Linking Research and Practice in Midwifery

For Baillière Tindall:

Publishing Manager: Inta Ozols
Project Development Manager: Karen Gilmour
Project Manager: Derek Robertson

Linking Research and Practice in Midwifery

A guide to evidence-based practice

Edited by

Sue Proctor PhD MSc RGN RM
Senior Nurse – Strategic Planning and Professional Development,
Bradford Health Authority, Bradford, UK

Mary Renfrew BSc PhD RGN SCM DN RN(Canada)
Professor of Midwifery Studies and Director, Mother and Infant Research Unit,
University of Leeds, Leeds, UK

Forewords by

Marc J N C Keirse
Professor of Obstetrics and Gynaecology, The Flinders University of South Australia,
Australia

Jennifer Sleep
formerly Professor of Nursing and Midwifery Research, The Wolfson Institute of Health
Sciences, Thames Valley University, Reading, UK

Jim Sikorski
General Practitioner, Lewisham, London, UK

Meg Wiggins Gready
Research Officer, Social Science Research Unit, Institute of Education, University of
London, London, UK

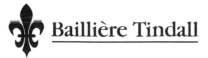
Baillière Tindall

EDINBURGH LONDON NEW YORK PHILADELPHIA ST LOUIS SYDNEY TORONTO 2000

BAILLIÈRE TINDALL
An imprint of Harcourt Publishers Limited

© Harcourt Publishers Limited 2000

✤ is a registered trademark of Harcourt Publishers Limited

The right of Sue Proctor and Mary Renfrew to be identified as editors of this work has been asserted by them in accordance with the Copyright, Designs and Patents Act 1988

First published 2000

ISBN 07020 2297 7

British Library Cataloguing in Publication Data
A catalogue record for this book is available from the British Library

Library of Congress Cataloging in Publication Data
A catalog record for this book is available from the Library of Congress

Note
Medical knowledge is constantly changing. As new information becomes available, changes in treatment, procedures, equipment and the use of drugs become necessary. The editors/authors/contributors and the publishers have, as far as it is possible, taken care to ensure that the information given in this text is accurate and up-to-date. However, readers are strongly advised to confirm that the information, especially with regard to drug usage, complies with the latest legislation and standards of practice.

The
publisher's
policy is to use
**paper manufactured
from sustainable forests**

Printed in China

Contents

Contributors

M. Rose Allen MAEd SEN SCM ADM PGCEA (MTD)
Rose Allen worked in the clinical field of midwifery for 13 years. Since 1983, she has worked in midwifery education. Presently, she is employed as a Senior Lecturer at the University of Leeds in the Division of Midwifery. Her responsibilities include integrating research into practice. Her main interests are related to midwives' continuing professional development. Rose is an active member of the editorial board for the *British Journal of Midwifery* and is the journal's special features editor. She undertook an MA in educational research at Lancaster University and is currently investigating the factors that influence midwives' continuing professional development.

Robina Aslam RGN RM PGCEA MSc
Robina Aslam has worked as a midwife since 1984 and has been active in midwifery education since 1992. She has taught at Greenwich and Sheffield Universities and is now Practice Development and Research Co-ordinator at St George's Hospital, South London. She completed her MSc in Inter-professional Health and Welfare Studies in 1995.

Debra Bick BA(Hons) MMedSci RGN RM FPCert
After obtaining a degree in history, Debra completed her nurse and midwifery training at hospitals in Birmingham. In 1992 she commenced a research post at the Department of Public Health and Epidemiology, University of Birmingham, to examine the extent, severity and effect of maternal health problems after childbirth. The study findings contributed to the successful funding of the trial she is currently working on, to evaluate a new model of protocol-based, midwifery-led, postnatal care. Her experience as the proud mother of twin daughters has contributed substantially to her research interests!

Angie Benbow BA(Hons) RN RM
Angie began her career in the NHS in 1974, training as a registered nurse in the first instance and moving to midwifery in 1980. Since qualifying as a midwife, she has developed a special interest in family planning and women's health issues in general. In 1995 she began working as a Research Fellow in the RCOG Clinical Audit Unit based in Manchester, on a number of joint and individual audit projects related to maternity care. As part of

the 'core' work within the unit, Angie jointly managed the RCOG audit help desk and database of clinical audit initiatives which reflects the audit culture in maternity care and gynaecology services across the UK. She now works as a Research Fellow with the Salford East Primary Care Group.

Elisabeth Buggins MHSM DipHSM
After professional training as a health services manager, Elisabeth left the NHS to look after three children with a variety of special needs. Whilst caring for them she worked with the voluntary sector on local, national and European projects. One example is the *Voices* Project which offered training and support to user representatives working with NHS maternity services. She has facilitated the interface between health professionals and users in many different arenas. Now chair of Walsall Community Health NHS Trust, and of Wolverhampton MSLC, she aims to build strong, multidisciplinary, multi-agency teams which work constructively to effect change. Her work with the voluntary sector continues.

Elisabeth Clark PhD BA(Hons)
Elisabeth Clark is currently Head of Distance Learning at the Royal College of Nursing (RCN) Institute. Although a psychologist by training, she has specialized in nurse education since the mid-1980s. Whilst at the Distance Learning Centre, South Bank Polytechnic, she was responsible for developing the first UK Diploma in Midwifery by distance learning, and also for the open learning research awareness programme for nurses, midwives and health visitors. This has sold tens of thousands of copies and sightings have been reported from all over the world, including in an isolated community health centre on a Greek island!

Soo Downe PhD MSc BA(Hons) RM
Soo Downe is currently the Research Midwife at Derby City General Hospital. She is responsible for the overall direction and management of the Maternity and Gynaecology Audit and Research Department at the hospital. She is also seconded to the local Health Authority to develop the long-term, collaborative, evidence-based strategy for the local maternity services. Her research interests include midwifery intrapartum practices, the evaluation of innovative maternity services, and the development of new methods in maternity services research, particularly in relation to application to practice.

Ray Field MPhil RGN RMN DipN(Lond) DipCPN CertEd RNT
Ray Field is Director of Nurse Education and Professional Development at St George's Health Care NHS Trust in South London. As chairman of the local nursing and midwifery research ethics committee and a member of the local research ethics committee he has reviewed a wide range of research proposals. He has contributed to conferences and training sessions for the pharmaceutical industry on ethics committee procedure.

Jennifer Hall MSc RN RM ADM
Jennifer Hall is a lecturer at the Mother and Infant Research Unit at the University of Leeds. She received clinical training and experience in Norwich and has also practised in a midwife-led unit in south west England. She has written a number of articles and has been involved with editorial work for the *Midwives Journal* in the *Nursing Times*. She has also been a manager at the Midwives Information and Resource Service in Bristol and was on the Council of the Royal College of Midwives. She has completed a Masters degree in Reproduction and Health. She is the mother of three small children (four by the time this is read!) and has a very patient husband!

Sue Hawkins BA DipLib
Sue Hawkins graduated with an honours degree in German but the only time this skill has been put to use since has been when attending various meetings of the German Midwives Association on behalf of MIDIRS. After university Sue took up a post as a Library Assistant in the Department of Community Medicine at St Thomas' Hospital in London, a Department of Health funded research unit. Following a year at the King's Fund Centre Library in London, Sue was appointed as MIDIRS's first member of staff in 1985 and was Information Services Manager until 1999.

Natalie Kenney BA MSc
Natalie joined the National Perinatal Epidemiology Unit (NPEU) as a project administrator in 1994. Owing to an interest in the research which the unit conducts, she undertook an MSc in Health Care Studies. For her dissertation, a qualitative approach was used to explore the reasons why pregnant women participate in midwifery-led, randomized, controlled trials. In her role as Researcher at the NPEU, she worked on a national survey of maternity units, health authorities and maternity services user representative groups to assess the extent to which maternity data are collected, disseminated and used. She is now a Researcher at the Ministry of Health, Queensland, Australia.

Hazel McHaffie PhD SRN RM
Hazel McHaffie has worked full time in research for the past fifteen years, leading a programme of work based in the University of Edinburgh in Scotland, but also participating in studies across Europe. Her principal interest has been the impact of events in Neonatal Intensive Care Units on families and health care professionals. Over the last seven years her focus has been on ethical issues, and alongside her empirical work, she campaigns to make ethics a user-friendly and clinically relevant subject. As part of that initiative she has written a novel, *Holding on?* which presents complex issues relating to decision making in an easily absorbed form accessible to lay and professional readers alike. She is the author of numerous publications and lectures extensively around the world.

Sally Marchant PhD RN RM ADM

After clinical midwifery experience of 9 years, Sally joined the NPEU in 1990 as Research Midwife to the Postnatal Care Project working with Jo Garcia. Her research to date has focused on practice related to postnatal care, using mainly survey research methods. She has just completed 3 years of study into routine assessment of uterine postnatal involution and vaginal loss by midwives in collaboration with Jo Alexander, Principal Lecturer in Midwifery Studies at the University of Portsmouth and Jo Garcia, Social Scientist, NPEU. She is currently involved in the NPEU's programme of work on unhappiness after childbirth and domestic violence in pregnancy, and works in clinical midwifery in her spare time.

Mary Nolan MA BA(Hons) RGN

Mary Nolan trained with the National Childbirth Trust (NCT) in the early 1980s. Since then, she has practised extensively as a childbirth educator both for the NCT and the NHS. For 5 years, she ran her own business mounting conferences for health care professionals and managers in maternity care. More recently, her commitment to childbearing women has been expressed through numerous articles in women's journals and the midwifery press and her first book entitled *Being Pregnant, Giving Birth* which appeared in 1996. Her PhD focused on empowering consumers through health education and has informed her third book *Antenatal Education: a Dynamic Approach*, published in 1998.

Sue Proctor PhD MSc RGN RM

Until recently, Sue Proctor was a Lecturer in Health Services Research at Guy's, King's and St Thomas' Medical School in the Department of General Practice and Primary Care. She completed her nurse and midwifery training in Manchester and Leeds respectively. After a period in clinical practice, she worked as research midwife for Bradford Health Authority on a large study examining the factors associated with birth outcome in Pakistani families. In 1994 she was awarded a NHS Research and Development (R&D) training fellowship which enabled her to study for her PhD, which was completed in 1997. She was appointed as Professional Editor for *Midwives*, the journal of the Royal College of Midwives in 1999. Sue continues to pursue her research interests in health care quality and involving consumers in assessing the quality of health care.

Mary Renfrew BSc PhD RGN SCM DN RN(Canada)

Mary Renfrew is Professor of Midwifery Studies at the University of Leeds, where she is also Director of the Mother and Infant Research Unit (MIRU). MIRU is a multidisciplinary unit, with research interests in the areas of inequalities in health, breastfeeding, and women's views of care and of research. MIRU works closely with colleagues in education and practice, to promote evidence-based care in midwifery. Before her move to Leeds in 1994, Mary was Director of the Midwifery Research Programme in the National Perinatal Epidemiology Unit for seven years. She worked as a midwife in Scotland and England, and taught and researched in Canada for several years, where she actively supported the legalization of midwifery. Mary was co-editor of the Cochrane Pregnancy and Childbirth Group, and still carries out Cochrane reviews. She sits on a range of committees for the NHS R&D programme, HEFCE, the Department of Health, and the MRC.

Michael Smith PhD MSc BSc CPhys FIPSM FinstP
Mike Smith is Dean of Research for the Faculty of Medicine, Dentistry, Psychology and Health, and Professor of Medical Physics at the University of Leeds. He is a member of the Central Research and Development Committee of the NHS, chairs the Diagnostics and Imaging Panel of the Health Technology Assessment Programme and was a member of the Culyer Implementation Group. He is the immediate Past President of the British Institute of Radiology, and Director of the Centre for Medical Imaging Research in the University of Leeds. He has many years' experience of multi-disciplinary research in university and NHS settings.

Ann Wraight RGN RM MTD PGCEA
Ann Wraight is the Quality Assurance Manager for the Women's and Children's Health Directorate at Pembury Hospital in Kent. The majority of her career has focused on midwifery – firstly as a clinical midwife in the UK and East Africa; then as a midwife teacher, manager in maternity and gynaecology services and, finally, as a research midwife before taking up her present post. She was the coordinator for three national studies – Pain relief in labour, Mapping team midwifery and Home births – and has also participated in research studies funded by the ENB and RCM.

Julie Wray MSc ADM RN RM ONC
Julie began her career in the NHS in 1974 and has experienced health care both abroad and in the UK. She worked as a midwife practitioner from 1981–1995. From 1995 to 1998 she worked as a Research Fellow in the Royal College of Obstetricians and Gynaecologists (RCOG) Audit Unit based in Manchester, on a number of joint and individual audit projects related to maternity care. As part of the 'core' work within the unit Julie jointly managed the RCOG audit help desk and database of audit initiatives.
Julie is currently writing her MSc dissertation based on a qualitative research study exploring midwives' attitudes towards screening for Down's syndrome. She is working as Research Fellow in the Health Care Practice Unit, University of Salford.

Gill Wright PhD BA(Hons)
Gill Wright is a Senior Lecturer at the Management Centre at the University of Bradford, where she teaches Consumer Behaviour and Marketing

Research. Her research interests focus on marketing in the public services, especially in health and social care. She is a member of the Chartered Institute of Marketing and the Market Research Society. She is a Visiting Fellow at the Nuffield Institute for Health in Leeds. Her interest and experience in research methods comes from a combination of collaborative research projects with health professionals, including midwives, as well as her role as Chair of the Doctoral Research Programme in Management and on the Executive of the European Doctoral Research Association.

Foreword

Marc J.N.C. Keirse
Care for pregnant women and babies has changed both drastically and rapidly in the last half of the twentieth century. It would be nice to state that midwifery has evolved along with or abreast of these changes. It is not true, though. Midwifery organizations have tended to follow evolutions in maternity care at so safe a distance that even the public at large recognizes change before they do. Of course, there are exceptions! The public should be pleased to see so much of their own philosophy reflected in the pages of this book.

Nevertheless, many people see little else than a midwifery profession lingering or languishing in self-indulgent reiterations of the 'with women' concept from which it derived its name. Clearly, there is nothing wrong with the name. Nor is there anything wrong with acknowledging one's roots. Names, however, should have meaning and roots should promote growth, not stunt it.

It would appear that midwifery spent so much time extolling the virtues of being 'with women' that it forgot how to be *for* women. Modern pregnant women, contrary to their predecessors and their peers in less fortunate parts of the world, can choose their own 'with women' persons. Not surprisingly, most choose partners, friends or relatives rather than 'with women' functionaries. After all, who has not come to realize that functionaries are of little value if they are only there *with* and not *for* you?

Obviously, 'for' is substantially more difficult to achieve than 'with'. It cannot rely on routines and traditions; nor can it be justified by any amount of jargon or self-righteous phraseology. However, as this book shows, 'for' is attainable.

This book may well be a signpost leading from the crumbling edifice of traditional midwifery to a tower of effective maternity care. It may be limited in its international perspective, but it certainly is not in the issues that matter to women here and elsewhere. Ethics matter and so do women's voices. Both found their way among the many other aspects that are vital to a profession that seeks to justify itself, rather than excuse or project its following. If this book promotes, as I hope it will, a midwifery profession that can justifiably act both with and for women, a major leap forward will have been made.

Marc J.N.C. Keirse MD DPhil DPH FRACOG FRCOG
Professor of Obstetrics and Gynaecology
The Flinders University of South Australia, 2000

Jennifer Sleep

Amongst current models of midwifery are two archetypes: midwifery as science and midwifery as art. We combine these in our imagination to create images of caring, sensitive practitioners who are able to use research appropriately to provide the very best of care. Each of these models is reassuring and comforting. They tell us that midwives will use their science to practise the most effective care and their art to recognize and meet women's individual needs.

Both models are useful but each has serious flaws. Often 'the art of midwifery' is based on assumption, clinical observation or personal experience; each of these impressions is potentially fallible, reflecting a worrying degree of what may be termed *unreliable certainty*. But, midwifery cannot be labelled as pure science because science is inherently reproducible and universal, and much of the research which helps us to understand the totality of the human experience reflects neither of these criteria. Yet research and development within the practice of midwifery has succeeded in reflecting both these models and, as such, is unique in health services research. This uniqueness stems from the different questions midwives ask which in turn spring from the privileged relationship they share with women, the richly diverse research traditions used to address issues and the creative strategies clinicians have developed to use research evidence to challenge and to change their practice.

This book offers unique and valuable insights into each of these aspects. Other texts have focused on the range of research methods which may be used to address the questions which arise from practice or have explored differing ways of achieving research-based care. But this is one of the first to explore the symbiosis which needs to exist between the conduct of high quality research and its subsequent use to inform the day-to-day decisions of both practitioners and policy-makers. This link between practice and its scientific base is essential if midwives are to be effective in providing women, their babies and their families with the very highest standard of care.

In the process, a number of important issues are explored from a range of perspectives. These include the relationship between education, policy and practice within an historical context, as well as current initiatives at both local level and across the health services as a whole. It provides a breadth of coverage and does not shrink from discussion of potentially contentious issues such as ethical dilemmas and the challenges which need to be addressed if women are to be honestly involved in setting the research agenda and in evaluating maternity services. It is only when we have access to a compilation such as this that we can piece together the jigsaw which reveals the whole picture of research in midwifery, its contribution and importance to the health and well-being of childbearing women and their families.

Jennifer Sleep, Professor of Nursing and Midwifery Research
The Wolfson Institute of Health Sciences, Thames Valley University,
Reading, 2000

Jim Sikorski

A recent survey of General Practitioners in Newcastle (Lipman 1998), the city where I trained, found that patients had presented 158 different problems in 413 consultations. The author of the survey suggests that clinical effectiveness will only be improved if the need for evidence to inform the management of this bewildering variety of problems is addressed. All health professionals face this particular, somewhat daunting, challenge – how to integrate the best available evidence into their daily practice. A text which sets out to be a guide to knowledge-based practice is, therefore, to be welcomed.

The task is complex – the path from research idea to efficiently delivered effective care is a long and tortuous one, which has been well sign-posted in this book. Despite these difficulties, the midwifery profession has already addressed the challenge in many areas with considerable success. The groundbreaking Midwives' Information and Resource Centre 'Informed Choice' leaflets have involved women in the final stage of this process.

In pursuing this important project of knowledge-based practice, however, all maternity care professionals might do well to heed my favourite quote from the Cochrane Library: 'Through seeking we may learn and know things better, but as for certain truth no man (sic) hath known it, for all is but a woven web of guesses.' The wise observation of a Greek philosopher, Xenophanes, in the sixth century BC!

Jim Sikorski, General Practitioner
Lewisham, London, 2000

Lipman T. 'Discrepancies exist between general practitioners' clinical work and a guidelines implementation programme' *British Medical Journal* (1998), **317**: 604.

Meg Wiggins Gready

If research into maternity care is done well, it can offer great benefit to women, their babies and their families. It is up to those of us who carry out research to do it to a high standard, with the needs of the participants clearly in our minds. This book offers midwives an opportunity to gain the necessary skills and to explore the relevant debates.

Users of the maternity services deserve to be offered care based on the best available research evidence. Health care providers and researchers know that a battle rages to make this common practice. Recent research carried out by the National Childbirth Trust (NCT) suggests that, while many maternity services users are not aware of the intricacies of research, most assume that their care is already based upon it. It is time to make their assumption a reality.

One of the key themes that you will find in this book is the challenge of involving the users of the service in all aspects of the research process. Most users welcome the chance to act as participants in research, for many appreciate the chance to share their experiences; to feel that what matters to them is valued by someone else as well. As one teenage mother said when asked to participate in NCT research, 'This is great. I feel really special. No one has ever cared what I think before'.

As well as an opportunity to talk about their experiences, many women consent to participate in research for altruistic reasons – they want to help others in the future. Users of the maternity services, as well as other users of health services, realize the need for research and so they consent to take part despite the fact that it may inconvenience them, or that the results may not ever have an impact on their own lives.

In addition to being involved as participants in research, users also have a role to play in shaping the priorities and nature of the research that is to be carried out. Chapter 5 of this book, 'Involving Consumers in Research' highlights the ways in which the involvement of users in these aspects can be invaluable. The challenges that researchers face in making users a key part of planning and implementation of studies can be far outweighed by the unique contributions that can come from such collaboration.

Users who are involved at any level, be it as a research subject or as a co-researcher, want to be taken seriously. They like be kept informed of progress and to see that results are being acted on. They want to see change as a result of their participation – or to be clear that the findings indicate that current practice is appropriate.

For many women, midwives are both their primary source of infor-mation on pregnancy-related topics and their only contact with health professionals. As such, midwives are uniquely placed, not only to carry out research, but also to disseminate research findings to women – to make results understandable and relevant. When attention to this aspect of the process is neglected, then it can undermine all of the work that has gone into an otherwise successful project. For example, in one health trust where there had been a recent policy change away from the routine practice of weighing women at antenatal check-ups, women using the services were unaware that the change had occurred because research had indicated that it was unnecessary. Instead they viewed the absence of a weight check as an omission based on forgetfulness or 'sloppiness'. The relationship that these women had with their midwives suffered as a result.

As *Changing Childbirth* (1993) highlighted the 'three C's' – choice, continuity and control – for women in maternity care, this book provides the necessary information for midwives to carry out crucial, competent, and collaborative research.

Meg Wiggins Gready, Research Officer
Social Science Research Unit, Institute of Education,
University of London, 2000

Expert Maternity Group *Changing Childbirth*, London: Department of Health 1993

Acknowledgements

We are indebted to many people who have worked with us to make this book a reality. Particularly, we would like to thank all the authors for their excellent contributions.

Very special thanks are owed to Charlotte Tomkies and Helen Bridges from the Mother and Infant Research Unit at Leeds University and Halima Miah from Bradford Health Authority for their exceptional secretarial support and patience throughout this project.

Introduction

Sue Proctor and Mary Renfrew

Midwives have a clear responsibility to ensure that the care offered to women and babies is based on the best available research evidence. This presents a number of challenges: for many aspects of practice, there is little or no evidence to support our decisions. For other aspects, however, information does exist, but still may not be used in practice to guide midwifery clinical decisions. There are many reasons for the gap between research and practice, but rather than focus on these, we should think about the risks of *not* using evidence to inform our care.

A fundamental principle of midwifery, and other health care professions, is *to do no harm*. This is the ethical basis of both clinical and research practice. However, it is important to recognize how, in the past, some interventions which were not based on evidence did more harm than good. These include routine inductions, routine episiotomies, restricting the mother's position at birth, taking babies away from their mothers on postnatal wards, and giving breast-fed babies top up feeds with formula milk. It is both challenging and uncomfortable to reflect on these and many other interventions which were once part of everyday practice, and the detrimental effects they may have had on women and their babies.

Midwifery is a challenging and a dynamic profession. Over recent years, midwives have demonstrated a commitment to developing and improving practice through research evidence and through a range of strategies for disseminating research findings, such as The Midwifery Research Database (MIRIAD) and the Midwives Information and Resource Service (MIDIRS). Through the development of an evidence-based culture (Renfrew 1997), midwives have worked hard to meet the challenges of providing woman- and baby-centred care which is based on the best available evidence.

Many questions about practice still remain unanswered. In addition, factors such as technological advances, changes in the way maternity services are organized, women's expectations of their childbirth experience and of what the service should offer, mean that there are still many issues, questions and challenges to be addressed. Because of these factors, midwives have to develop their knowledge on a continual basis, learn new things and keep moving forward.

Striving to develop and improve our practice starts with asking questions about what we do for women and babies. Finding answers to our questions may involve reflecting on particular events, reviewing the literature, or conducting a research study ourselves. Then we have to identify whether there is a need to change practice, implement that change and to continue to improve and develop our knowledge and clinical care.

This book is written for midwives to help them meet these challenges, and to support them, not only to find answers to questions about practice, but also to use their findings to inform and guide the continuing improvement of care provided to women and babies.

Why do we practise in a particular way?

In the real world, it is often difficult to take a step back from the busy clinical area, whether this is a home, health centre or hospital, to ask this question. However, if we want to understand why we practise in a certain way, and then to support our decisions with evidence which will enable us to account for our actions, then it is a question which is too important not to ask.

Many midwives and students are familiar with the process of reflection, as they learn and develop their knowledge and experience. After registration, we may reflect less. Sometimes, it is not until we are faced with a new experience or are working in a new practice area, that we start to reflect, not just on *why* we practise in a certain way, but why we had never *questioned* it before. By thinking about our practice and reflecting on the effect it has on women and babies in our care, we can identify gaps in our knowledge and areas where we need to develop. Box 1 illustrates an example.

SOURCES OF MIDWIFERY KNOWLEDGE

For many aspects of midwifery practice, there is little or no research evidence available to support clinical decision-making, although for many others there *is* information which is not put into practice. Not all aspects of practice require a base of *research* evidence, however. For example, we don't need to test if women prefer to be cared for by courteous and polite staff.

Some aspects of practice are based firmly on our experience and competence, which develop over time. For example, the discussion which takes place between a midwife and a woman about which position is best for the birth will be influenced by many factors. Knowledge of research, the mother's preference and the experience of the midwife will all contribute to the outcome of the discussion. Midwifery knowledge, and, consequently, practice is influenced by a number of sources and these are illustrated in Figure 1.

EVIDENCE-BASED PRACTICE

We considered using the term *'knowledge-based practice'* rather than *'evidence-*

Box 1   Why do we practise differently?

Julie was a midwife who worked part-time, usually 2 nights a week. She had been qualified for 8 years, and had had a 2 year break when she gave birth to her daughter. She moved to a different part of the country and had been at a new maternity unit only 3 weeks. This was her first night in the labour ward. It was a relatively quiet night and Julie worked with Samina, a midwife who trained at this unit.

Samina was caring for Claire, a primagravida at term, who was doing well in labour. Claire soon progressed towards full dilatation. Both midwives stayed with Claire and supported her during the second stage of her labour. Julie watched while Samina advised Claire that she could push when she felt the urge. With each contraction, Samina waited for Claire to push and encouraged her with a 'well done' when she paused for breath.

Julie felt frustrated. With each contraction she wanted to tell Claire 'to put her chin on her chest, hold her breath and push hard'. Surely the baby would be delivered more quickly and it would all be over. This was the first delivery Julie had attended for almost 2 years, and she felt anxious, partly because she was concerned for the fetus and Claire, but also for herself. She knew exactly what she would normally say at this stage, but Samina was letting Claire just get on with it. Julie felt like a 'spare part'.

Julie's mind was full of questions. Do all the midwives here just let the women push when they like? What if Claire didn't progress? How would they explain not encouraging active pushing to the doctor? Does this actually do any good? Does holding the breath make a difference? Surely it must be right, we've done it for years? Within 40 minutes or so, the baby's head was visible and soon afterwards Claire gave birth to Luke, a healthy 3.5 kg boy.

Fortunately, as it was a quiet night Julie was able to ask Samina many of the questions she had and they discussed the issue of active versus spontaneous pushing. Samina said she had read that getting women to hold their breath and push for long periods might actually be harmful, tiring them out, and may have a detrimental effect on the oxygen supply to the fetus. She also said that a study had found that 'breath holding' pushing only shortened labour by a small amount. If women felt more in control by pushing spontaneously, and the fetus was okay, then to her, letting them push spontaneously seemed a reasonable thing to do. Julie made a point of going to the library to read up on this aspect of practice, because she wanted to know if she should change her practice and why.

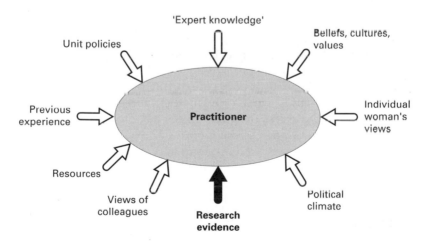

Figure 1   Influences on decision-making in midwifery

based practice' in this book, to acknowledge the range of influences on clinical decisions in midwifery. The term 'evidence' can sometimes be interpreted in a narrow way and may be associated only with findings from well-designed, randomized and controlled trials. Whilst such research is recognized as the gold standard, in reality, a combination of factors influence our decisions and interventions for individual women and babies in our care. The key point is that if good evidence is available, it should be used to inform our practice. Sackett et al (1996) provide a useful definition of evidence-based medicine which incorporates these important issues:

'Evidence-based medicine is the conscientious, explicit, and judicious use of current best evidence in making decisions about the care of individual patients. The practice of evidence-based medicine means integrating individual clinical expertise with the best available external clinical evidence from systematic research.'

Given the incorporation of different sources of knowledge in this definition, the term 'evidence-based practice' describes the care we believe to be important for women and babies. Evidence-based practice, ideally using knowledge derived from good quality research, matters throughout every aspect of the care provided to women and babies. It should be the basis for:

1. the information given to women as they experience pregnancy and childbirth
2. the support for women as they care for themselves and their babies
3. all midwifery, nursing, medical and therapy provision
4. the organization and delivery of maternity care
5. the cost effectiveness and clinical effectiveness of that care
6. the organization and delivery of health care services, and the continuing development in terms of the quality of those services.

The impact of knowledge on effective practice has far reaching consequences. This includes contributing to safety and clinical effectiveness in maternity care around the world. Dissemination of such knowledge is of global importance. In many parts of the world, women and babies die as a consequence of inadequate or poor care during pregnancy and childbirth. There are huge variations, not only in the care given to women and babies, but also in the access their caregivers have to information and the knowledge that is shared across the world. For example, episiotomy rates vary internationally from 80% in Argentina, 33% in Botswana, to 20% or less in England (Maduma-Bushe et al 1998).

Evidence-based practice is at the centre of high quality maternity care. There is an ethical imperative to deliver care which is based on the best available information, to minimise the risk of doing harm (Hazel McHaffie discusses this important issue in Chapter 4). As a concept, it embraces research findings, knowledge gathered through professional and life experiences, and an awareness and understanding of women's preferences about their care.

Steps to evidence-based practice

Questioning our practice, and that of others involved in the care of women and babies, is only the first step in beginning to develop evidence-based midwifery care. Box 2 presents a range of questions which midwives might ask about practice.

Seeking answers to those questions is the next step. When we start to look for answers to our questions, we may find a number of different scenarios (Figure 2).

Answers to questions may be found in some of the excellent resources which focus specifically on pregnancy and childbirth research. In Chapter 6, Jenny Hall and Sue Hawkins discuss these resources, and what they can offer midwives. They include *Effective Care in Pregnancy and Childbirth* (Chalmers et al 1989), the *Cochrane Library* (1998) and the Midwifery Research Database, MIRIAD (McCormick and Renfrew 1998). These resources provide an opportunity to access a range of high quality research evidence.

If, as for Julie in the story in Box 1, the answers to our questions exist and are both accessible and understandable, this information can be used to inform practice. Research is useful in informing us about what should be done because it is beneficial, unrestricted breastfeeding for example, or what should no longer be done because it is harmful, such as using glycerol impregnated catgut for suturing the perineum. In Chapter 8, Soo

---

Box 2 Questions about practice

What is the ideal number of routine antenatal visits?
Why are women given so much information at the booking appointment? Why isn't it more evenly distributed over their pregnancy?
What advice should be given to women who want to do aerobic exercise during pregnancy?
Why in some units do women have a routine cardiotocograph (CTG) for 20 minutes when they are admitted in labour? Why 20 minutes?
Why do some midwives suture any tear whilst others will not suture skin tears? Does it make a difference to the woman's healing or discomfort?
Some women are permitted to eat and drink during labour, but others can only have water. What are the risks and benefits of these practices to mother and fetus?
What are the risks and benefits of active versus expectant management of the third stage in primiparous women?
What differences are associated with different cord care practices?
How many routine postnatal visits are ideal?

These are only examples. Think of questions about your area of practice. How much of what you do for women and babies is based on research evidence?

Evidence exists ➡ can answer your question ➡ can be used to inform and support practice ➡ discuss with colleagues/manager ➡ implement change as necessary ➡ audit practice ➡ continue to develop practice and improve quality.

Evidence exists ➡ possibly can answer your question ➡ can't be sure it is good quality research or sufficient as base to change practice ➡ identified learning need ➡ research appraisal skills ➡ take action.

Evidence exists ➡ possibly can answer your question ➡ can't get access to it due to:

- lack of time ➡ negotiate with manager/colleagues/midwifery educators
- library hours too restrictive ➡ inform librarian/ask manager to do likewise
- don't know how to use computer databases ➡ find out about local training at the library or education centre
- library doesn't stock relevant journals ➡ inform librarian/manager and educators/ find out about using inter-library loan services.

Evidence does not exist in midwifery literature ➡

- Can other sources of knowledge help?
- Talk to midwifery/medical/other professional colleagues.
- Do you know what women's views are?
- Do they think it is important?

Think about conducting a research study ➡ where will you seek advice/ support ➡ review relevant literature ➡ think about your research question ➡ think about and plan a research study ➡ talk to others about your ideas ➡ get expert advice ➡ what are the ethical issues? ➡ design a research proposal, think about and plan every aspect of the study ➡ obtain ethical committee approval ➡ conduct your study ➡ disseminate the findings, locally and in publications/conferences ➡ influence and inform practice.

Figure 2   Possible pathways from asking questions about practice

Downe discusses the issues around dissemination and implementation of evidence.

It may be that such findings help to support current practice, or suggest that change is needed. Audit is a useful tool for monitoring whether the right thing is being done and for helping to develop practice standards based on research evidence. Julie Wray and Angie Benbow discuss the important contribution of audit to midwifery practice in Chapter 9. Knowledge developed though the audit process can be further supported by keeping up to date with the most recent evidence, through reading professional journals regularly, attending conferences and study days or taking part in other educational activities. In Chapter 10, Rose Allen presents some of the key issues in midwifery education and continuing professional development.

Research can sometimes leave us in a sort of limbo, when we learn that there is not enough evidence to indicate whether a practice is either of benefit or harmful, such as giving birth in water. These discoveries are very important as they help us identify the questions that we still need to find answers to. This means that we can develop the evidence base of our practice without reinventing the wheel.

Using high quality research evidence as a basis for clinical decision-making lies at the centre of evidence-based practice (Renfrew 1997). However, not all published research is of the same quality. Being able to understand research evidence, and to distinguish poor from good quality research requires important skills that all midwives should possess. Even among good studies, there is a hierarchy of quality to consider when thinking of applying research findings to practice (Box 3).

Sometimes, information exists which can answer our questions but, for a range of reasons, it is not accessible. This may be due to a lack of relevant journals in the local library. Access may also be limited if the library is only open 'office hours' which are not compatible with shift working. A huge amount of research is published electronically and access will be affected if the Internet or certain databases are not available locally. Access to literature held on computers is also compromised if we do not have the skills and knowledge to find our way around the software. Time constraints may be a big problem, particularly for those working in the community, who may have to make a special trip to a hospital library in a rare lunch break or in their own time after work.

For some topics, particularly new procedures, such as the impact of screening tests in early pregnancy, or older procedures which are new to midwifery, such as the effects of aromatherapy in labour, there may be very little information. Conducting a research study may be the only way to reach an answer to our question.

Box 3   Hierarchy of evidence

1. Evidence obtained from at least one properly designed, randomized, controlled trial
2. a) Evidence obtained from well designed, controlled trials without randomization
   b) Evidence obtained from well designed cohort or case-control analytical studies, preferably from more than one centre or research group
   c) Evidence from comparisons between times or places with or without the intervention – dramatic results in uncontrolled experiments could be included in this section
3. Opinions of respected authorities, based on clinical experience, descriptive studies or reports of expert committees

Source: Baker & Kirk 1998

STRUCTURE OF THE BOOK

This book aims to provide an opportunity for midwives to explore and understand the fundamental relationship between research and practice. It is structured in two sections. The first, and largest section presents a series of important chapters which discuss strategic and contextual issues around using research to develop evidence-based care in midwifery. The second, shorter section presents a series of brief chapters, which aim to provide an introduction to the core skills of doing research in midwifery.

Section One

Section One can be described in three closely related parts. The first focuses on the context of midwifery practice, its use of research evidence, interactions with other professions, and its relationship with the wider research and evidence-based agenda in health care. The second builds on issues raised earlier and takes us through some key stages of developing evidence-based practice. The final chapters discuss approaches to continuing the development and improvement in midwifery practice.

The context of midwifery practice

The book begins in practice, starting with a discussion by an experienced clinical midwife on the role and importance of research in midwifery practice. The implications of research on clinical decisions, and issues of professional accountability and risk management are analysed. These are illustrated with many practice-based examples.

Chapters 2 and 3 then broaden the discussion. Firstly, the history and significance of research in the development of midwifery practice is examined. The evolution of research in midwifery, and its future challenges and directions are highlighted.

The importance of the development of practice based on research evidence is a theme throughout the whole NHS. Chapter 3 discusses the links between midwifery and the wider research community. It discusses the significance of the NHS Research and Development Strategy, and the opportunities for midwives to influence research priorities, gain research funding, and to use this initiative to further develop practice.

Developing evidence-based practice

Chapters 4 and 5 address important gaps in the current literature. They each discuss critical steps in the planning and thinking phases of research, which are often taken for granted. Ethical issues are an important part of planning and conducting research, as they are in the decision to implement research findings in practice. Based on the principles of doing good and minimizing harm, Chapter 4 discusses the importance of ethics in midwifery practice and research for midwives who are clinicians, researchers or managers.

We are aware of the importance of involving women in decisions about their care, but how can we involve them in the process of developing evidence-based practice? Chapter 5 discusses this crucial issue. Ways of identifying and addressing the priorities of women and babies are analysed and suggestions are given for involving them in every stage of the research process.

Chapters 6, 7 and 8 take a closer look at the key stages of the process of developing evidence-based practice. They are not intended as comprehensive guides to research methods, as interested readers are well served by an extensive range of specialist publications on research philosophy, methodology and analysis.

The key elements in the process of conducting a literature review of a practice issue are discussed in Chapter 6. This includes the use of existing data sources, and the skills required in critical appraisal of published papers. Chapter 7 provides a clear analysis of the need for matching appropriate research methods to research questions. With a range of examples from many aspects of practice, this chapter helps dispel some of the mystique around the research process.

The findings of research studies, or of literature reviews can present many challenges and opportunities. They may confirm existing practice or suggest the need for urgent change. Approaches to managing the dissemination of research findings, and their application to practice are discussed in Chapter 8 in this section. This shifts the focus very clearly back to clinical practice.

Continuing to develop and improve evidence-based practice

The next set of chapters tackles issues around how we can monitor what happens in practice to ensure that it continues to be based on research evidence. Chapter 9 discusses the process of developing standards for care. The role of clinical audit in midwifery and its contribution to developing quality care is also analysed. In addition to developing our practice, individual professional development is essential. Chapter 10 unites the themes of practice, research and education and discusses how they interact.

The book began in practice, is packed with practice-related examples and illustrations, and, in Chapter 11, includes a transcript of a group discussion of clinical midwives. They discuss the contribution of research to their practice, factors which help in delivering evidence-based care and those which hinder its development. They discuss where they see the future of midwifery research and practice and how these elements contribute to each other. Chapter 12 provides a summary of this section and also looks forward into the future.

Section Two

Some midwives may find their questions about practice cannot be answered sufficiently by reviewing existing knowledge. In such cases, it may be appropriate to consider conducting a study which can help provide an answer. This section does not attempt to provide a comprehensive research methods guide, as many other excellent resources exist which meet this objective. However, in five relatively short chapters some of the core skills for someone starting to conduct research in midwifery are discussed by experts in the field. In each case, examples are provided for the reader which may help them improve and refine their project. These include designing a research proposal and applying to a research ethics committee. Some methodological principles are also presented. Research approaches which are popular in research in midwifery are examined, such as designing a questionnaire, conducting an interview and conducting observational research. Guides for further reading are also included in each of these brief chapters.

Consistent themes

Throughout the book there are a number of important themes which link the discussions around research, evidence-based practice and quality of care:

1. Research and the development of midwifery knowledge should be driven by practice. As answers emerge to research questions which derive from practice situations, whether from systematic reviews or new research, they should be widely disseminated to practitioners.

2. Understanding research papers and being able to judge the quality of published studies prior to using findings to inform practice are essential midwifery skills.

3. Midwives do not practise in a vacuum, and should be aware of national R&D policy and research priorities, including how these affect maternity services. The importance of collaborating with other professionals in developing research and practice is emphasized.

4. Women and babies demand a quality service and, as accountable professionals, we need to justify our interventions with good evidence whenever possible. Research shouldn't be done *on* women and babies, but *with* them. Their involvement – as with care – should be active. Addressing their priorities for research *and* practice enables them to become active contributors, not passive 'subjects' in research studies and in the development of maternity services.

5. Providing evidence-based care requires a passion for continual improvement in practice and professional development.

ONE LAST THING ...

Our interest in research involving women and babies has its roots in clinical practice. Coming from quite different experiences of midwifery, we both wanted to find out more about why we, as midwives, practise in a certain way. Topics we have examined include perineal care, understanding more about women's experiences of breastfeeding, the effectiveness of the care and advice they are offered, what women want from maternity services, why particular groups of women are more likely to have a poor birth outcome, and what interventions may reduce risk. Working with women and babies, other midwives, general practitioners, obstetricians, paediatricians and many others, we have learnt that research can be stimulating, frustrating, exciting, hard work, rewarding and fun – just like midwifery!

REFERENCES

Baker M, Kirk S *Research and Development for the NHS*, Second edition Oxford: Radcliffe Medical Press; 1998
Chalmers I, Enkin M, Keirse MJNC *Effective Care in Pregnancy and Childbirth* Oxford: Oxford University Press; 1989
McCormick F, Renfrew MJ *MIRIAD Register* Third edition Hale, Cheshire: Books for Midwives Press; 1998
Maduma-Bushe A, Dyall A, Garner P 'Routine episiotomy in developing countries: Time to change a harmful practice' *British Medical Journal* 1998; **316:** 1179–80
Renfrew MJ 'The development of evidence based practice' *British Journal of Midwifery* 1997; **5:** 100–104
Sackett DL, Rosenberg WMC, Gray MAJ, Haynes BR, Richardson SW 'Evidence-based medicine: what it is and what it isn't: It's about integrating individual expertise and the best external evidence' *British Medical Journal* 1996; **312:** 71–72

The context of midwifery research and practice

This section comprises 12 chapters which allow the reader to explore a range of issues associated with the key relationship between research and practice. It begins with a discussion of the contextual issues. Developing clinical practice, building on the historical development of research within midwifery, developing new and strengthening existing partnerships with other professions all support the link between research and practice. It is also helpful to consider research and development in the context of the NHS as a whole. Ethical practice is as important in clinical activity as it is in research. Similarly, working *with women* is an essential part of each stage of the research process, as in clinical practice. These issues are discussed comprehensively.

Thinking about why we practise in a certain way – asking questions about practice and about any evidence which may underpin it – can lead to a number of actions. Reviewing existing knowledge, designing a research study to answer our questions, and using the knowledge from these processes to inform and change practice involve a range of skills and abilities. Subsequent development and improvement require that we address the challenges of practice and professional development. Clinical audit and education are key tools to enable such challenges to be met.

The section ends with a discussion by practising midwives about their experiences of using research in practice. This and the final chapter reflect on the many themes raised in the earlier chapters and present a framework for the future to develop and sustain the links between research and practice.

1

Research and evidence in midwifery practice

Robina Aslam

KEY ISSUES

- What is 'research'?
- What is 'evidence-based care' and how does this relate to research?
- What are the advantages and disadvantages of research and evidence-based care in midwifery?

- How are research and evidence-based care perceived by midwives and other allied professionals?
- How is evidence-based care implemented in practice?

INTRODUCTION

Linking these various strands together is part of the move towards a new clinical culture which emphasizes evidence and is called 'evidence-based care' or 'evidence-based practice'. A number of factors have fostered this development. Modern technology has meant that staff must constantly update themselves, rather than relying on techniques learned during their training. Growing awareness by women and interest groups, such as the National Childbirth Trust (NCT) and Association for Improvements in the Maternity Services (AIMS) have encouraged the development of staff. The profession itself has sought improved status for its members leading to undergraduate training for all recent trainees. A spin-off from this has been that students have acquired critical skills and have not been content to follow procedures without question. This, in turn, has encouraged all staff to adopt a more reflective approach to their practice.

A major milestone in these developments in the UK was the *Changing Childbirth* report (Department of Health 1993) which highlighted the fact that many practices were not supported by evidence. It suggested that midwives should be able to appraise new developments critically and provide sound up-to-date information for women and their babies in order for them to make informed choices about their care.

Nevertheless, many midwives remain sceptical and unconvinced about the need for evidence-based practice. This chapter aims to explore the issues described above and to confirm that using the best available evidence when planning care in partnership with women is a fundamental part of the role and responsibility of every modern, safe midwife.

Box 1.1 Reflection activities

Consider the following:

- What does 'research' mean to you?
- What does 'evidence-based practice' mean to you?
- Must midwives be 'researchers' to be effective clinicians?
- What do you feel has been the impact of research on clinical practice?
- In what ways has the philosophy of 'evidence-based practice' changed clinical practice?
- How may research affect practice in the future?
- Identify research evidence which has influenced your practice.

Before reading further, ask yourself the questions posed in Box 1.1. They will be discussed in this chapter, but take a few minutes now to reflect on what they mean to you.

RESEARCH IN MIDWIFERY

In order to be able to place the points made in this chapter into the right context, it is worth spending a few minutes referring to the brief overview set out in Box 1.2.

The nature of research

The concept of learning through research is an ancient one. Historically, in science and medicine research has played a key role in developing our understanding of anatomy, biochemical processes, pharmacy and clinical procedures. Such research took a variety of forms including:

- dissection, observing the location and function of organs
- analytical tests, for example, on placental cells to develop an understanding of the processes involved in the physiology of the placenta
- trials to determine the principal effects and side-effects of drugs e.g. ergot.

The uniting factors behind these different types of research are (a) methodical observation and (b) the development of a theoretical model which is (c) developed and refined over a period of time. For example, in the case of anatomical dissection, the position of and relationship between the perineal body and perineal muscles is observed in a number of cadavers so that an understanding of 'normal' structure can be determined, leading to a model of normal anatomy. In the case of physiology, the understanding of the process of wound healing enhances effective care management.

Box 1.2   An overview

- **What is 'research'?**
  Research is the collection and analysis of data in a systematic manner.
  For example, a midwife may wish to determine whether average birthweight for term babies is related to maternal age. After discussion with a statistician, birthweight data could be collected for babies at term and plotted on a graph against maternal age to see whether there is a correlation. Such a plot will give a primary indication. More conclusive research would require the use of statistical tests to determine whether associations, which appear at first sight to be correct, may be proven – for example there are likely to be very few births to mothers over 50 years old and so it may be wrong to draw generalizations from the small amount of data available.

- **What is 'evidence-based care' and how does this relate to research?**
  Evidence-based care is the use of evidence in making decisions about the care of individual women.
  Evidence comes in a variety of forms. The best evidence is that obtained from high quality research programmes, such as those using randomized, controlled testing and series of fully-documented case histories. Such evidence is, however, not always available; here midwives may use their own experiences which have been carefully noted and reflected upon. The key is always to use *the best* evidence available. The expression 'evidence-based care' suggests that decisions based on tradition alone are often unsound; for example enemas and shaving were at one time universal, as a matter of tradition, until research showed that they were generally of no effect.

- **What are the benefits (and drawbacks) of research and evidence-based care?**
  Research and evidence-based care ensure that decisions are taken on the basis of clinical effectiveness, rather than past experience. This is of benefit to mothers, babies and staff who aspire to act professionally. The drawbacks include the fact that not all aspects of practice have a research evidence base, and it is not always realistic when dealing with snap decisions, such as an obstetric emergency.

- **How are research and evidence-based care perceived by midwives and other allied professionals?**
  The leaders of the midwifery profession accept the value both of research and evidence-based practice. Recently qualified midwives will understand the benefits as this will have formed part of their studies. Amongst midwives of longer standing, there are some who recognize the benefits and are enthusiastic about the opportunities presented by research and evidence-based care, whilst others have not yet been convinced. It must be accepted that midwives must improve their research skills if aspirations for collaborative working are to be realized.

- **How is evidence-based care implemented in practice?**
  The key moment at which evidence-based care is required is when decisions are to be made about the programme for delivery and intervention. This process interacts strongly with the process of 'risk management' since particular programmes of treatment do not necessarily lead to particular outcomes, but influence them. For example, research may show that vaginal delivery of term breech presentation babies results in a fetal death rate of 1%. This information helps inform the decision-making process but cannot determine what individual decision is taken.

The development of research in midwifery

Historically, midwifery has differed from many other areas in the medical arena in that research in the above sense has *not* been the principal source of procedural developments. The reasons for this are many and complex. They include the following:

- Childbirth is a natural process and, unlike medical intervention, predates historical records. Childbirth processes were in use long before any concept of learning by systematic observation had been developed.
- Childbirth, like other events associated with reproduction, has always been surrounded by taboos and myths, many of which are more dependent on cultural, emotional and social factors rather than physical factors. Many of these remain today.
- Historically, the existence of a class of people (traditionally women) without scientific qualification of any type, yet deemed qualified to act as midwives, enabled a range of procedures to develop based on tradition without any reference to efficacy.

Recently, the evidence-based culture has been applied to midwifery practice with good effect (Renfrew 1997). Thus, for any procedure, even one which has been used since time immemorial, it is now proper to ask: Why are we doing this? Is it effective? Is there some other procedure which is more effective? Examples include questioning the efficacy of routine pre-delivery enemas and use of Savlon for postnatal perineal care. It was found that both procedures were ineffective and simply served to waste time, resources and potentially undermine the dignity of women (Romney & Gordon 1981, Sleep & Grant 1988).

Research must, of course, be justified in terms of its benefits. Some of these are set out in Box 1.3.

Types of research in midwifery

Research is not only about questions which have yes or no answers. Indeed, some of the more important questions addressed by researchers are those in which risks are quantified. For example, a midwife presented

---

Box 1.3 Justifications for research in midwifery

- Women and babies deserve evidence-based care.
- Midwives are able to identify areas of midwifery practice where more, or better, evidence is needed.
- Midwives are ideally placed to become involved in programmes in which clinical effectiveness is examined.
- Midwives can provide a link between women and policy-makers and hence need to understand research policy.
- Midwifery is rapidly developing as the lead profession in normal delivery and must take on the associated responsibilities.
- A common research philosophy assists in the development of inter-professional collaboration.

with a fetus lying in a breech position may wish to know what the risk of mortality is. This information can be obtained from the analysis of statistics from a large number of births containing both breech and other positions. From these data, the absolute and relative risks associated with the fetus lying in different positions can be ascertained. It is easy to see, however, that simple analysis may often lead to misinterpretation. For example, the mortality rates such as still birth rate (SBR) or perinatal mortality rate (PNMR) may change over time or from country to country and, therefore, a mixture of data from different dates and places may give a misleading picture.

Although the concept of research is relatively simple to understand, the proper conduct of research may require the application of sophisticated statistical analysis and other procedures to disentangle the various factors which may distort the proper conclusions.

Errors may be introduced into the data because the people being observed respond to the fact that they are being observed (the Hawthorne effect). For example, during a drug trial in which some people are given the treatment and some are not, the participants' responses may be significantly affected by their expectations of the drug's likely efficacy. In order to prevent this, drug trials are often conducted 'blind': some participants receive 'control' placebos and some receive the test drug. This largely avoids this problem. However, experiments can often be influenced by the *researcher* knowing which participants are taking the drugs and which are taking the placebos and so 'double-blind' trials are used for the highest level tests. These are trials where even the person administering the treatment does not know whether the subject is receiving the test drug or a placebo (randomized double-blind controlled testing).

Although randomized controlled testing is designed to eliminate the preconceptions and perceptions of the subject and observer from the equation, much valuable research in the field of midwifery is precisely *about perceptions*. Women from different social or ethnic groups may respond differently to different procedures carried out, for example, giving colostrum as a first feed. Such procedures may be acceptable to women from one social group but wholly unacceptable to women from another group. Likewise, information which is readily understood by one group may, for reasons of language or culture, not be understood by another. Since midwifery is about women-centred care, the perceptions of women are crucial to the performance of professionals and hence have to be understood through research rather than guessed at.

In many cases, simple research procedures yield obvious insights; for example, asking 10 women, randomly selected from a literate social/ethnic group, to what degree they understand a leaflet designed to inform them. If their overwhelming response is that they do not understand the leaflet, then complex discussions about statistics become irrelevant. The fact is that a significant proportion of women do not understand the leaflet and it has to be rewritten.

In other cases, complex statistical analyses are important, as is the adoption of criteria for ranking results. Imagine two distinct schemes of perineal care, A and B, applied to women with the same class of trauma. The recovery is rated Poor, Moderate, Good and Excellent, and the results from tests on 200 women, 100 of whom received each care, yield the following results:

Table 1.1   Results from an investigation into perineal care

Scheme of care	Poor	Moderate	Good	Excellent
A	5	38	44	13
B	0	44	56	0

The first question is: are these results significant or do we need to do more tests to ensure that the results are sufficiently representative? This is a question for a statistician. The second question is: which treatment is the 'better' treatment? This is a question for a policy-maker because it depends on the definition of 'better'; different people may well propose different definitions and women themselves may have a different approach to, say, a midwife or a doctor.

The above discussion demonstrates that a wide range of research types and techniques are relevant to midwifery. Some involve simple, easy-to-understand techniques; some require the assistance of statisticians and other specialists.

Evidence-based care

Evidence-based care has been defined as 'the conscientious, explicit and judicious use of current best evidence in making decisions about the care of individual patients' (Sackett et al 1997). At its root is the idea that decisions must be made about each woman individually, based upon the evidence available.

Hierarchies of evidence are described by a number of writers (e.g. Rosenberg and Donald 1995). One possible ranking of the hierarchy of evidence is given in Box 1.4 (see also page 7).

Evidence-based care relies upon evidence *used appropriately*. There are a number of key ideas involved and these are demonstrated in Figure 1.1. This figure implies that there is a hierarchy not just of evidence as suggested above but also of objectives. The hierarchy of objectives is given tentatively and the types of objectives that the various participants may hold are illustrated in Box 1.5.

In general, the higher the evidence type in the hierarchy, the greater the weight it should be accorded. However, even when good quality research

Box 1.4 Hierarchy of evidence

1. Randomized controlled testing
2. Controlled testing on selected groups
3. Non-controlled testing
4. Testing on selected small samples
5. Evidence from tests carried out outside a formal research environment
6. Personal experience
7. Clinical tradition
8. Anecdotes.

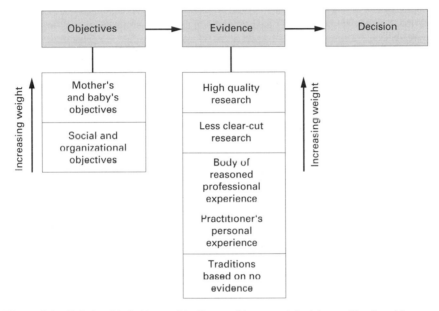

Figure 1.1 Relationship between objectives, evidence and decision-making in evidence-based care

data are available to assist decision-making, the midwife should use all evidence in its proper context; all available evidence means research findings, clinical experience, clinical skill and judgment as well as the preferences of women.

Furthermore, that use must be explicit; in other words, midwives must be able to explain their decisions, identifying the evidence used to inform them.

Objectives in midwifery practice

Clearly any decision must be based, first and foremost, on the objectives we are seeking to achieve. If we are not clear about these, we will not know

---

Box 1.5 Objectives in midwifery practice

The principal objectives of midwifery must be determined collectively as a matter of policy. It is suggested that a typical professional midwife sees the role in accordance with the following objectives:

- supporting the successful birth of a viable child
- advancing the long-term quality of life of the child
- promoting the physical well-being of the mother
- promoting the emotional well-being of the mother
- preserving resources which may be valuable for others requiring care
- avoidance of claims for negligence and/or trespass.

Note that this list of objectives is derived from the consideration of a number of perspectives. For example the objective of procuring the successful delivery of a live baby is generally the principal objective of the mother and the midwife, and always of the child; it protects the interests of the organization as well. The objective of avoiding claims is clearly an objective of the organization and the midwife.

Each of these objectives is, of course, not always consistent with all other objectives. For instance, a woman who presents with a breech pregnancy may be advised that in terms of risk to the baby, a caesarean section is the safe option. However, many women experience negative emotional and physical effects following a section delivery (Reid 1993, Wood 1992). In such cases, the objectives conflict and the risks have to be assessed in terms of the multiple, competing objectives.

---

which evidence is relevant. These points are best explained by examples and two are presented below. The first example demonstrates the types of issues which may arise when there are multiple, competing objectives. The second involves a decision which is fairly representative of those which midwives must take in practice. In both examples, fabricated evidence is used for purposes of illustration.

Example one

A term fetus presents as a breech and the following three pieces of (fabricated) evidence are available:

1. The risk of the breech baby's death during a vaginal delivery is 1% and only 0.1% during a caesarean.
2. The risk of serious perineal tearing during vaginal birth is 10%, while physical and emotional trauma during caesarean is about 20%.
3. The cost of a caesarean is twice that of a vaginal delivery and prevents access to a bed, perhaps by a woman with a more serious condition.

Assuming that one accepts these (fabricated) data as accurate, both vaginal and caesarean birth entail risks. One is unable to decide upon the appropriate course of action until the relative weight to be applied to each objective is known. Assuming that the survival of the baby is the key objective to which all others must be sacrificed, a caesarean section is the correct decision. However, in real practice, the decision is sometimes taken to commence vaginal delivery, monitor the situation closely and be prepared to go for emergency section if the need arises. This provides a sound balance between the various objectives.

Example two

During delivery a woman suffers second degree perineal trauma. The midwife is undecided whether or not to suture. The following factors appear relevant:

1. There is some anecdotal (i.e. undocumented but considered reliable) evidence that perineal healing following a moderate tear is adequate, despite leaving the perineum unsutured (Yiannouzis 1998). There are also some sound experimental findings (Gordon et al 1998) which suggest that leaving skin layers unsutured is no more likely to result in problems than complete suturing. This evidence may, by extrapolation, support the anecdotal evidence.

2. During a study carried out by a sister on the ward as part of her MSc degree, the average times for suturing procedures were: 15 minutes preparation; 20 minutes suturing; approximately 10 minutes post-suture care.

3. The cost of absorbable suturing materials is about £10.

This example illustrates a typical decision which a midwife faces. The primary objective is to produce the best healing of the trauma, and this is readily broken down into sub-objectives.

1. Woman's objectives:
   - the fastest repair
   - alleviation of pain
   - most effective repair with the maximum post-repair function
   - avoidance of unnecessary intervention (i.e. the initial suturing or subsequent removal of stitches)
   - short-term and long-term peace of mind.

2. Midwifery/organizational objectives:
   - completion of the total care for the woman, including consideration of both short-term and long-term outcomes
   - to minimize resources (i.e. time occupying beds, midwives' time, material costs)
   - to minimize risk of post-repair problems which may involve additional resources and – in extreme cases – legal action.

The midwife is required to weigh and balance these objectives. In terms of weight, the midwife may decide – following consultation with the woman – that the key objective is the 'maximization of post-repair function' and that all other sub-objectives must give precedence to this one (in fact, many of the others follow from this, such as long-term peace of mind and minimizing risk of legal action etc.). Even if this simple approach is adopted, there is the problem that the evidence upon which to base the judgment is unclear; while suturing appears effective, there is no evidence that *not* suturing leads to negative outcomes and may actually be beneficial, as well as saving resources. If the midwife decides to suture using absorbable materials, then, given the current state of the evidence, that decision cannot be considered as other than professional. Deciding not to suture would be questionable on professional grounds, as well as leaving the midwife open to legal action. Nevertheless, this example highlights the need for evidence to be made available from high quality research in order to inform decisions and to enable midwives to practise with confidence.

So, as seen in Figure 1.1 and in the examples developed, the two stages prior to making a decision are:

1. understand the objectives
2. understand the evidence available.

Having achieved this level of understanding, a midwife can proceed to make a rational decision which can be justified in the particular circumstances of the case. This is evidence-based care.

BENEFITS AND RISKS OF RESEARCH AND EVIDENCE-BASED CARE IN MIDWIFERY

Spend 15 minutes on the following exercise (Box 1.6).

The benefits of evidence-based care

Evidence-based care potentially benefits the woman, the baby, the midwife and the employer, as shown in Figure 1.2. This figure shows that interaction is neither one-way, nor restricted to specific parties; it is relevant to

---

Box 1.6 Group exercise

- Identify a practice issue or procedure which you feel is not based on research evidence.
- How and why do you think this practice was adopted as part of routine midwifery care?
- What are the benefits of this practice for the women and babies? Who else benefits from this practice?

Keep a note of your discussions as these will be developed further in later chapters of the book.

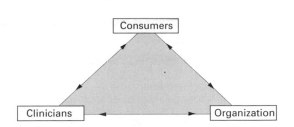

Figure 1.2   Beneficiaries of evidence-based practice

the entire process of care and creates the basis for an inclusive, inter-professional approach in which women's objectives are discussed with them and the interests of all parties are weighed and taken into account. This is consistent with the change in the philosophy of childbirth care over the past few years. It has moved away from an expert-centred approach, with midwives and obstetricians providing expertise and exercising control, to a woman-centred approach in which the woman is a full and active partner in the process. Indeed, consumer groups and other sources now provide women with details of the latest research findings which may affect their pregnancy and birth and, as a result, many women are well-informed. Many women would be most disconcerted to find that their midwife is unaware of the implications of the latest research. It is no longer a luxury for midwives to be informed about the latest research, but an integral part of the information-giving and pastoral aspects of their job, as well as central to their clinical role.

The key benefits of evidence-based practice to the main stakeholders are summarized in Box 1.7.

Benefits to the mother

For the mother, evidence-based care means that she receives care which is informed, tested for its benefits and tailored to her particular circumstances. In addition, she is encouraged to become a member of the decision-making team and she is informed of the procedures and their purposes. The decision-making process depends fundamentally upon the objectives which are sought; as discussed, the objectives which the mother specifies must be taken into account. Any decisions may impact upon the mother and baby's quality of delivery – and sometimes quality of life – and informed consent for any intervention is imperative. Therefore, the involvement of the woman in the decision-making process is vital. This is recognized in current NHS policy (*Changing Childbirth* Department of Health 1993) and is fostered by evidence-based care. An example is the administering of Vitamin K to neonates; women are advised about the advantages and potential problems associated with administering this to their babies.

Box 1.7 Advantages of evidence-based practice

Advantages for women and their families:

- up-to-date information and openness
- involvement in decision-making processes
- increased options of care based on available evidence
- improved quality through the abandonment of ineffective or harmful practice
- adoption of effective and beneficial practices
- areas identified where improvements can or should be made
- resources directed to the appropriate women
- dissemination of evidence encourages standardization of good practice.

Advantages for professionals:

- produces reflective, confident, assertive midwives
- provides basis for constructive debate about practice developments
- enables midwives to develop professional autonomy
- enables inter-professional teams to operate more effectively.

Advantages for organizations:

- enables resources to be managed more effectively
- promotes improved standards of care and quality
- development of competent workforce
- promotes standardization and greater efficiency.

Benefits to the midwife

Midwives have aspired to the position of lead professionals in normal childbirth (i.e. the vast majority of cases). However, midwives must, by the same token, recognize that, if they are to benefit from full professional status, they must also be prepared to defend their practice rationally. This means that they must be aware of the research base and be able to evaluate it critically. Once this status is achieved, it will result in a profession empowered to empower women and respected by other professionals, as well as one which takes pride in constantly improving the level of its care. More generally, research is intellectually stimulating and creates a body of motivated and committed professionals, enabling them to participate in the development of their own field. Research awareness encourages midwives to develop and participate in innovations in practice and increases confidence in the decision-making process.

Benefits to the organization

It is in the interests of the health care organization for midwives to work efficiently and effectively, applying valuable resources where they can be best used, without subjecting women and babies to undue risk or otherwise causing negligent harm. Increased research understanding means increased quality, which will impact upon efficiency, innovation and service delivery. Hospitals benefit when professionals collaborate on the basis of a shared research understanding, rather than on the basis of their own individual traditions. Research findings enable midwives to consider the best allocation of their resources. Thus, by identifying the risk factors for women in pregnancy, more antenatal care can be provided for those who need it without increasing the overall workload. Likewise, the judicious and explicit use of research and risk management strategies based on evidence reduces the likelihood of errors, as well as providing sound reasoning to answer claims for negligence. Inter-professional collaboration improves team work and co-operation in formulating guidelines and policies.

Examples of the benefits of research and evidence-based care in midwifery. The following examples illustrate the value of evidence-based care in changing practice.

- Examples of effective procedures which have been introduced:
  - agents to reduce stomach acidity in labour
  - external cephalic version at term
  - pain relief such as epidurals
  - new suturing materials.
- Examples of comforting procedures which have been shown, by research, to be safe:
  - support in labour
  - mobility and position in labour.
- Examples of ineffective procedures which have been abandoned:
  - sodium bicarbonate solution for resuscitation
  - enemas before labour
  - shaving before labour
  - salt baths
  - routine use of powder for cord care
  - routine episiotomy
  - antenatal nipple preparation
  - perineal sprays
  - restrictions on breastfeeding
  - routine electronic fetal monitoring.
- Procedures which are currently used but which are being investigated:
  - routine inductions
  - routine ultra sound
  - caesareans upon breech presentation
  - vitamin K to neonates
  - hydration in labour.

For more detailed information on these and other practices, see Enkin et al (1995).

Evidence-based care: the downside

So far, the emphasis has been upon the positive aspects of evidence-based care. In order to take a balanced view, it is important to appreciate the problems too.

The principal concern relates to the perceived conflict between research and individualized care. Many people feel that the introduction of decisions based on 'efficacy' will erode the traditional role of the midwife in offering individual care, tailored to the needs of the woman. However, evidence-based care in midwifery care does not mean that a midwife must override a woman's preference in planning care. Instead it should allow the woman and the midwife together to take responsibility for the planned action of care.

There are also real concerns about the implementation of evidence-based care; three problems immediately present themselves:

1. The cost of evidence-base care
2. Resistance to change
3. Urgent decision-making.

The cost of evidence-based care

The use of evidence in midwifery care carries a cost. There is the cost of research, the cost of teaching students and midwives how to utilize the techniques of evidence-based care and the time required by midwives to analyse practical situations as they arise. However, the hope is that, as research funding becomes more widely available and the profession becomes more and more research-aware, the benefits in terms of improved efficiency of caring for women and babies, the removal of ineffective processes and the reduction of damage and litigation will more than pay for the investment.

Resistance to change

As with every cultural change, there will be resistance. This will arise as a result both of (a) the normal reluctance of people to change practices which they feel have been operating successfully for many years and (b) midwives' fear and lack of confidence in their ability to consider and assess research evidence.

Urgent decision-making

When a woman (or baby) needs urgent care, it is not always convenient or possible to obtain guidance from research. In these situations, professionals rely on clinical judgment and experience. Some of this may be informed by research and it is to be hoped that, as the research base improves and dissemination of evidence to practitioners increases (e.g. through audit, risk management, reviews etc.), these judgments will be based increasingly upon sound evidence.

PERCEPTIONS OF RESEARCH AND EVIDENCE-BASED CARE BY MIDWIVES AND OTHER ALLIED PROFESSIONALS

The development of research and evidence-based care relies on a number of factors including a positive perception on the part of midwives that research is important. The UKCC (1993) states that 'midwives must advise and support women and their families during childbirth. They must be up to date in their knowledge and support their practice with evidence'.

Changing Childbirth (Department of Health 1993) recommended that midwives should take the lead role in midwifery care and, as such, every practitioner has a duty to be able to base their practice on the best available evidence. This is supported by consumer groups such as NCT and AIMS which are involved actively in conducting, participating in and disseminating research.

Traditionally however, many midwives have been trained on practical courses with little emphasis on academic rigour. The focus was often on traditional methods with the belief that accumulated wisdom produced the best care and greatest comfort for mother and baby; when difficulties arose, the delivery was handed over to an obstetrician. As a result of this lack of research training and awareness, many practising midwives feel uncomfortable with research. Most new graduates have undertaken small research exercises as part of their studies and have some knowledge of critical appraisal techniques, and so are more confident in reading and assessing the quality of published studies and such concerns may not apply to this class of midwife (Storer-Brown 1997).

Harris (1992) found that midwives rarely used research evidence to inform practice. Hopefully, now this picture is changing. The latest information from the MIRIAD Midwifery Research Database (McCormick and Renfrew 1998) indicates a significant rise in the number of registered midwifery research projects. In 1996, 426 midwifery research studies were noted. In the third edition (1998), 29 new studies were registered and to date 53 new studies have been registered. These figures suggest that research in midwifery is being undertaken and that the findings are welcomed by an ever increasing proportion of the profession. Nevertheless, the total proportion of the midwifery profession who participate in research studies remains low.

Attitudes

A significant number of empirical studies have been carried out to determine the attitudes of midwives and other healthcare professionals to research. Generally, they conclude that many have resistant attitudes to research (for example, Hicks 1996). The term 'researcher' appears to many to denote a different set of qualities to 'clinician': a study by Hicks (1995) suggests that 'a midwife who is categorized as a good researcher may be perceived as a poor midwife and vice versa'. However, these findings need to be put in their temporal context – there has been increasing interest in research even since this study was undertaken. Focus group work undertaken locally indicated that amongst a mixed-age group of midwives, there was an increasing understanding of the value of research, even if the results of this study may have been affected by peer pressure or concern that the midwives should be seen to support hospital policy.

Confidence

One of the key issues in any attempt to introduce a research culture into midwifery practice is that midwives should feel confident in reviewing research findings. Many midwives feel they do not have the skills to appraise research findings critically and accurately (Meah et al 1996). Some are no doubt correct to a degree. It would be a monumental task, of course, to retrain all midwives to have a deep understanding of statistics, experimental design and so on. However, evidence suggests (Hicks 1994) that significant improvements in both skill and confidence levels can be obtained from more limited training sessions, such as short study days.

Midwives as researchers

Surveys conducted in the early 1990s showed that midwives who undertake research are slow to publish because of diffidence (Hicks 1993) and that midwives are less confident in the ability of other midwives to carry out research than they are of obstetricians. This is also supported by the numbers of registered midwifery projects in MIRIAD. Again, these surveys were carried out some time ago and the results may be less marked today. The low confidence of midwives is likely to be reinforced by the low opinion of midwives' views held by some doctors (Hunt 1987).

Barriers

Many midwives believe that there are barriers to the implementation of research. These include accessibility of libraries at the time of need and the technical language of research publications (Lacey 1994, Meah et al 1996).

In addition, during a focus group study conducted locally, some midwives saw research as an extra burden when time resources were already limited. This is backed up by research by Kajermo et al (1998), who suggested that a lack of colleagues with whom to discuss work was a problem, but that the appointment of a specialist midwife with research qualifications would facilitate the improved research understanding of midwives generally. Lacey (1994) indicated that nurses (and the same may be true for midwives) did not feel sufficiently confident to challenge their work colleagues. Parker (1994) proposed that they were not reading the right articles. Renfrew (1997) suggested that they were unable to find all the relevant published material and, indeed, there are many aspects of midwifery practice for which no sound research exists (Page 1996). Much research is seen to be irrelevant to practice (Renfrew & McCandlish 1992) and the priorities need to be identified (Sleep et al 1995).

Addressing the barriers

Despite these difficulties, it is important that research is seen as part of the normal midwifery process. One way to do this may be to alter the way in which midwives make clinical decisions (Gray 1997, Sackett et al 1997). Where decisions are considered in the light of the risks and opportunities associated with any course of action, decisions cannot be justified on the basis of historical precedent but only on the basis of effectiveness. Working in this way necessitates a critical approach and familiarity with current research. There is a shift in the burden of proof; no longer do researchers have to justify their role to the clinician, but the clinician has to justify to women her reluctance to understand the latest evidence. This decision-making process can be enforced by documentation procedures which state reasons for courses of treatment as well as what happened.

Training days in research methods and periodic presentations of the latest findings in a variety of areas will reinforce the sense that research is important and relevant to day-to-day practice (Proctor 1996). Barriers such as terminology are gradually being overcome as more midwives begin to publish work for their peers. Access to libraries and journals has also improved.

Midwives should be encouraged to reflect critically upon their own practice. This is not to say that they should experiment on women; but, at the same time, they should not forgo the opportunities to develop a fund of empirical information which may – within the limits of ethical considerations – be used to inform practice. Certainly, the existence of researched practice and treatments in midwifery is limited and it is simply not possible to base all evidence on controlled trials alone.

In some sense, many midwives are already research active; they play a vital role in assisting with sample collection (for example, placental and blood samples) and questionnaires. However, they rarely become involved in the analysis of data or see projects through to publication.

PRACTICAL IMPLEMENTATION OF EVIDENCE-BASED CARE: THE WAY FORWARD

The successful implementation of evidence-based care in midwifery requires support and resource commitment by the organization. Gray (1997) suggests: 'The organization's structure should promote and facilitate evidence-based decision-making ... for any organization to increase the degree to which decisions taken within it are evidence-based, it is important to develop the right systems and culture.' Page (1997) goes further, suggesting that evidence-based care in midwifery requires a change in the power distribution and organization of care.

Indeed, professionals working within any structure must play their part in encouraging and influencing changes. Many organizations already function within this framework, for example regular audit meetings, implementation of risk assessments, clear evidence-based policies and guidelines and journal clubs all contribute to the ethos of research and evidence-based midwifery. However, research (Berggren 1996, Kajermo et al 1998) suggests that midwives lack confidence in applying findings to practice. Midwives felt a need for practice development led by a specialist. In recent years, posts for practice development and research midwives have become common and this shows the commitment of organizations to this approach. The effectiveness of such initiatives has yet to be evaluated but, based on anecdotal information, they provide support and encouragement for midwives. Nevertheless, many midwives will not have access to such specialist support; accordingly organizations will need to develop strategies for improving skills in the area of evidence-based practice in alternative ways.

These points will be discussed in more detail in later chapters of this book.

CONCLUSION

This chapter has introduced the basic concepts of research and evidence-based care in midwifery. It has examined the image of research within the profession and highlighted the need for midwives to use – and in some cases to carry out – research to inform their practice.

Within the next decade a number of factors will mean that the value of research will become almost universally accepted in the profession. The majority of practising midwives will be educated to degree level; managers will encourage midwives to develop themselves using research; furthermore, midwives will need to work inter-professionally on the basis of a shared research understanding and with the increasing involvement of women in active care planning.

If midwives aspire to be the lead professionals for routine childbirth, they will have to become accountable for the decision-making process in the planning of midwifery care. They must be accountable. This requires an understanding based on the evidence and research.

FURTHER READING

Lockett T *Evidence-based and cost-effective medicine for the uninitiated* Oxford: Radcliffe Medical Press; 1997
   This book is aimed at health care professionals with little or no prior knowledge of the subject. It is a useful guide.
Crombie I K *The pocket guide to critical appraisal* London: BMJ Publishing Group; 1997
   This extremely useful, pocket-sized book provides the reader with valuable assistance in interpreting research evidence.

REFERENCES

Berggren AC 'Swedish midwives' awareness of attitudes to and use of selected research findings' *Journal of Advanced Nursing* 1996; **23:** 462–470
Department of Health, *Changing Childbirth – Volume 1* London: HMSO; 1993
Enkin M, Keirse MJNC, Renfrew MJ, Neilson J *A Guide to Effective Care in Pregnancy and Childbirth* Oxford: Oxford University Press; 1995
Gordon B, Mackrodt C, Fern E et al 'A randomised evaluation of two stage postpartum perineal repair leaving the skin unsutured' *British Journal of Obstetrics and Gynaecology* 1998; **105(4):** 435–440
Gray JA *Evidence-based Healthcare. How to make health policy and management decisions* London: Churchill Livingstone; 1997
Harris M 'The impact of research findings on current practice in relieving postpartum perineal pain in a large hospital' *Midwifery* 1992; **8:** 125–131
Hicks C 'Rallying midwife researchers: how to increase output' *British Journal of Midwifery* 1993; **2:** 89–95
Hicks C 'Bridging the gap between research and practice: an assessment of the value of a study day in developing critical research reading skills in midwives' *Midwifery* 1994, **10(1).** 18–25
Hicks C 'Good researcher, poor midwife: an investigation into the impact of central trait descriptions on assumptions of professional competencies' *Midwifery* 1995; **11:** 81–87
Hicks C 'Nurse researcher: A study of a contradiction in terms' *Journal of Advanced Nursing* 1996; **24:** 357–363
Hunt J 'The process of translating research findings into nursing practice' *Journal of Advanced Nursing* 1987; **12:** 101–110
Kajermo KN, Nordstrom G, Kruseebrnat A, Bjorvell H 'Barriers to and facilitators of research utilisation as perceived by a group of registered nurses in Sweden' *Journal of Advanced Nursing* 1998; **27:** 798–807
Lacey EA 'Research utilisation in nursing practice – a pilot study' *Journal of Advanced Nursing* 1994; **19:** 987–995
McCormick F, Renfrew MJ *MIRIAD Register* Third edition Hale, Cheshire: Books for Midwives Press; 1998
Meah S, Cullum C, Luker A 'an exploration of midwives attitudes to research and perceived barriers to research utilisation' *Midwifery* 1996; **12:** 73–84
Page LA 'The backlash against evidence-based care' *Birth* 1996; **23:** 191–192
Page LA 'Evidence-based practice in midwifery: a virtual revolution?' *Journal of Clinical Effectiveness* 1997; **2(1):** 10–12

Parker C 'breastfeeding: research and quality assurance issues.' *British Journal of Midwifery* 1994; **2(2):** 56–60

Proctor SR *The development of research in practice* The first annual midwifery and neonatal nurses conference, University of Northumbria, 1996

Reid T 'Cutting decisions' *Nursing Times* 1993; **89(40):** 16–17

Renfrew MJ 'Influencing the development of evidence-based practice' *British Journal of Midwifery* 1997; **5(3):** 131–134

Renfrew M, McCandlish R 'With women – new steps in research in midwifery' in Roberts H *Women's Health Matters* London: Routledge; 1992

Romney ML, Gordon J 'Is your enema really necessary?' *British Medical Journal* 1981; **282:** 1269

Rosenberg W, Donald A 'Evidence-based medicine; an approach to clinical problem solving' *British Medical Journal* 1995; **310:** 1122–1126

Sackett DL, Richardson WS, Rosenberg W, Haynes RD *Evidence-based medicine: how to practice and teach EBM* London: Churchill Livingstone; 1997

Sleep J, Grant A 'Effects of salt and Savlon bath concentrate postpartum' *Nursing Times* 1988; **84(21):** 55–57

Sleep J, Renfrew MJ, Dunn A, Bowler U, Garcia J 'Establishing priorities for research; report of a Delphi survey' *British Journal of Midwifery* 1995; **3:** 323–331

Storer-Brown D 'Nursing education and nursing research utilisation: is there a connection in clinical settings?' *The Journal of Continuing Education in Nursing* 1997; **28(6):** 258–262

UKCC *Midwives Rules* London: UKCC; 1993

Wood M 'The unseen scars' *New Zealand College of Midwives Journal* 1992; **6:** 18

Yiannouzis K Abstract writer's comments on the MIDIRS review of 'The Ipswich Childbirth Study: 1. A randomised evaluation of two stage postpartum perineal repair leaving the skin unsutured' *MIDIRS* 1998; **8(3):** 339

2

The historical context of research in midwifery

Elisabeth Clark

KEY ISSUES

- Background and context of the early development of research in midwifery
  - Towards a 'research-based' profession
  - The contribution of social scientists
  - The role of the National Perinatal Epidemiology Unit (NPEU)
    Some early midwife-led research studies and the Midwifery Research Initiative
  - The move of midwifery education into higher education

- The first doctorates awarded to midwives
- The emerging pluralism of research in midwifery
  - The contribution of different research perspectives
  - An analysis of methodology
  - The distinctiveness of naturalistic methodologies
  - Achieving greater clarity in research in midwifery
  - Lay perspectives in research in midwifery
- The way ahead.

INTRODUCTION

Within this chapter I aim to provide an overview of the growth of research in midwifery over the past 20 years or so and to illustrate the advances being made by midwives towards the development of a sound knowledge base for maternity care.

Any such analysis must be influenced by the particular perspective of the author. As a psychologist (my academic background) and someone who, since the mid-1980s, has been concerned with promoting research awareness in both nursing and midwifery rather than actually doing research, I must be classed as an outsider. Potentially, this status brings with it the advantage of some degree of detachment, but the associated disadvantages of not being fully aware of the latest discussions that may be occurring within the midwifery research community. Whilst my analysis will inevitably be partial, it is intended to stimulate debate about the research infrastructure within midwifery, and the extent to which midwives are well placed to take up the opportunities offered by the NHS Research and Development (R&D) strategy (1991).

BACKGROUND AND CONTEXT OF THE EARLY DEVELOPMENT OF RESEARCH IN MIDWIFERY

To appreciate the development of research in midwifery requires a broad understanding of the health services context – in particular, the evolution of the NHS R&D strategy and the associated drive towards evidence-based health care. These and other important contextual issues are addressed in more detail in Chapter 3. If you have not read this chapter, you are advised to read it now before proceeding any further.

Without research evidence it is difficult to differentiate between un-substantiated prejudice and reliable knowledge. The following quotation identifies, implicitly at least, concerns about effectiveness and cost that permeate much health services research activity today and it sums up the health care climate of the late 1990s:

'It ought to be a matter of genuine concern – to patients [in the case of midwifery this means childbearing women and their babies], health professions, politicians and taxpayers – that there is little, and often no scientific basis for much of the health care which is delivered under the name of the National Health Service. Instead of high quality research, the factors which dictate the content of much clinical practice are subjective or even subliminal. Most of what we do, we do because we do it; history, tradition, obscure and often personal notions of professionalism and unsubstantiated opinion continue to dominate too high a proportion of decision-making in health care. This ... applies to all the key professions in the field.' (Baker 1998)

This quotation echoes earlier assertions by leading figures such as Chalmers (1989) and Peckham (1991), and highlights one of the key driving forces behind the launch of the NHS R&D strategy in 1991. The *Changing Childbirth Report* of the Expert Maternity Group also found that 'tradition plays a large part in the way maternity care is organized. The Group saw a good deal of evidence that practice was not always based on measures known to be effective' (Department of Health 1993a).

Towards a 'research-based' profession

If we go back more than 25 years and refocus on specific developments within nursing and midwifery, then perhaps one of the earliest milestones was the publication, in 1972, of the Report of the Committee of Nursing. This wide-ranging report included a phrase which has since become a near mantra – namely that 'nursing should become a research-based pro-fession ... a sense of the need for research should become part of the mental equipment of every practising nurse and midwife' (Department of Health and Social Security 1972). Later in this document the word 'should' changes to 'must'. As we shall see, these paragraphs influenced strategic thinking in nursing and midwifery over the next two decades, and, as a consequence, there has been a steady movement towards midwifery knowledge and practice becoming informed by research findings. Whilst this chapter will explore specific steps along this journey, this entire text and, indeed, other recent midwifery publications provide impressive evidence of what has been achieved to date.

Even before 1972, however, there were some examples of research studies in nursing, most notably the work of early pioneers such as Lisbeth Hockey and Marjorie Simpson. As Nursing Officer (Research) at the Department of Health and Social Security (DHSS), Simpson was responsible for setting up 'The study of nursing care' research project, in 1967, in collaboration with the Royal College of Nursing. This major project launched the research careers of six nurses through one of the earliest research training programmes in nursing (McFarlane 1970), and was followed by annual DHSS Research Fellowships which enabled more nurses to undertake research and enrol for research degrees.

The contribution of social scientists

However, prior to the mid-1970s, the concept of a research basis for midwifery practice had not really been on the agenda and there were certainly no midwifery-led projects on the scale of, or of equal importance to, the one mentioned above. Research into maternity care was largely undertaken by obstetricians working within a medical model of care. Some important research was, however, being carried out by social scientists. For example, Kitzinger's early descriptions of parents' emotions during childbirth (Kitzinger 1971), women's experiences of induced labour (1975) and of breastfeeding (1979); Oakley's work on becoming a mother (1979, 1980); Cartwright's study of childbearing and induction (1979); and the work of Tew (a statistician) which demonstrated that mortality rates for home births were no higher than those for hospital births (Tew 1978, 1979) despite widespread assumptions to the contrary and the specific recommendations of the Peel Report that all women should have a hospital confinement (Standing Maternity and Midwifery Advisory Committee 1970).

It could be argued that this early social science research laid the foundation for the broad research base that now characterizes the research undertaken by midwives today. Right from the start, the views and experiences of women have been regarded as centrally important, thereby challenging the medical model of maternity care with its emphasis on cause and effect relationships and the effectiveness of forms of care, often at the expense of listening to women themselves and acknowledging their experiences. Research such as that undertaken by Tew also highlighted the need to challenge existing practices through the analysis of routinely collected data – a trend that has continued through one of the 'strands' of research activity undertaken at the National Perinatal Epidemiology Unit (Macfarlane & Mugford 1984, Macfarlane et al 1995).

The role of the National Perinatal Epidemiology Unit (NPEU)

Against this background of a dearth of research in midwifery, the establishment in 1978 of the NPEU (a multi-disciplinary research unit within Oxford University) was a crucial initiative. With Iain Chalmers (an obstetrician) as its first director, this unit has provided an important focus for multi-disciplinary research in the perinatal field within the UK – a focus that continues to this day. In 1998, its core staff included a social scientist, an epidemiologist, an economist and a medical statistician, and together with the project staff, there were 10 different disciplines providing that all-important mix needed to undertake multi-disciplinary research.

The aim of the NPEU, which was core funded by the then DHSS, was to 'provide information which can promote effective use of resources in the perinatal health services' (NPEU Report 1991). It is interesting to note that this aim offers a foretaste of what was to become the thrust of the first NHS R&D strategy some 12 years later, except that the latter's focus encompassed the entire health services. It is also, perhaps, no coincidence that the earliest major collection of systematic reviews of research evidence underlying alternative forms of care was published in the perinatal field (Chalmers, Enkin & Keirse 1989). These reviews were subsequently incorporated into the Cochrane Collaboration Pregnancy and Childbirth Database, and, more recently, within the Cochrane Library. Since the late 1980s, therefore, midwives have had access to some of the best collations of research evidence of any health care specialty (see Chapter 6).

The NPEU's impact should not only be assessed by its research output – an impressive measure in its own right, with 853 publications and 49 NPEU papers and reports between 1978 and 1997 – but also by its outreach activities. During these early years of establishing research in midwifery, important work was undertaken by the unit staff in providing support for inexperienced researchers, giving lectures and running workshops, offering assistance with writing research proposals, responding to enquiries, providing advice to those undertaking or who were considering undertaking perinatal trials (the Perinatal Trials Service) and sitting on national committees. Without such a focus of excellence and expertise, it would have been more difficult to support those midwives wishing to undertake research. Although the NPEU was, perhaps, the most obvious national focus of research support for midwives at the beginning of the 1980s, there were other avenues including universities offering research supervision and encouragement.

Two editorials in 1991 acknowledged the contribution and expertise of the NPEU and both the national and international influence of its work (Young 1991, *The Lancet* 1991). Moreover, a formal review of the work of the unit (as part of the Department of Health's review of all its funded research units) acknowledged that 'the scientific quality of the NPEU's work was of national and international standing. The Unit is a world leader in perinatal research' (NPEU 1994). Despite this outstanding academic achievement, those associated with the NPEU could never be accused of being 'ivory-tower' academics: close collaboration with clinical colleagues and users of the maternity services has always been a hallmark of all their research activity. This is a feature that is mirrored in much research in midwifery today.

As would be expected, most of the staff employed in the NPEU during its early years are now working elsewhere, taking with them invaluable experience and extensive research networks. Indeed, their dispersion has contributed significantly to the continuing development of perinatal research as they continue to push forward the research agenda in a number of different institutions throughout the UK.

Some early midwife-led research studies and the Midwifery Research Initiative

Two of the earliest, best-known studies led by a midwife investigated evidence of the effectiveness of the routine procedures which most women disliked intensely. Romney conducted trials on perineal shaving (Romney 1980) and the use of enemas (Romney & Gordon 1981) which have since been instrumental in changing midwifery practice and in eliminating a major source of discomfort for thousands of women in labour.

In 1988, the NPEU provided the home for the first major externally funded research programme in midwifery to be headed up by a midwife, Mary Renfrew – the Midwifery Research Initiative. However, well before this initiative, several midwives had approached the NPEU with specific ideas for research which then led to joint projects. In 1981, Jennifer Sleep, at that time a midwifery tutor, proposed a randomized controlled trial on the effects of restricted versus liberal use of episiotomy. The idea behind this study emerged directly from clinical practice: as a midwife she had become intrigued by unsubstantiated claims that the liberal use of episiotomy offered advantages for women and their babies. The results of the West Berkshire Perineal Management Trial were published in both the *British Medical Journal* and *Nursing Times* (Sleep et al 1984, Sleep 1984a, 1984b). However, had it not been for the support of researchers at the NPEU, this trial might never have got off the ground. Collaboration with colleagues, particularly the epidemiologist, Adrian Grant, enabled a midwife to work alongside researchers from other disciplines and learn a great deal in the process (Sleep 1985).

Adrian Grant also collaborated with Jean Proud (Head of an Obstetric Ultrasound Service) on a trial into the use of third semester placental grading by ultrasonography as a test of fetal well-being (Proud & Grant 1987). Between 1983 and 1988, Sally Garforth was employed as a research midwife to work on a large-scale study of policy and policy-making in midwifery care in English health authorities (Garforth & Garcia 1987, 1989, Garcia et al 1987, Garcia & Garforth 1989). These early studies were funded or part-funded by the DHSS, charitable trusts such as Iolanthe and Birthright, regional health authorities, and also by research scholarships offered by the Royal College of Midwives in conjunction with Maws. Core staff at the NPEU clearly played a significant role in this early phase by enabling a small nucleus of midwives to conduct research.

Sleep's initial research on episiotomy led to a series of trials, each addressing an important aspect of perineal care. These included a follow-up after three years of the episiotomy study (Sleep & Grant 1987a); a controlled trial of glycerol-impregnated chromic catgut with untreated chromic catgut for the repair of perineal trauma (Spencer et al 1986) and a follow-up study of dyspareunia associated with the use of glycerol-impregnated chromic catgut (Grant et al 1989a); a trial of pelvic floor exercises in postnatal care (Sleep & Grant 1987b); a randomized controlled trial to compare the routine addition of salt or Savlon bath concentrate during bathing in the immediate postpartum period (Sleep & Grant 1988); and a randomized placebo-controlled trial of ultrasound and pulsed electromagnetic energy treatment for perineal trauma (Grant et al 1989b). This entire series of trials led by a midwife is reported in Sleep (1991). Following extensive consultation with both individuals and groups involved in maternity care, the Midwifery Research Initiative (MRI) focused initially on three main areas:

1. The systematic evaluation of midwifery practices in common use (the MAIN trial: multicentre trial of alternative treatments for inverted and non-protractile nipples in pregnancy).

2. The use of research in practice (the development of the Midwifery Research Database (MIRIAD) to record ongoing and completed research in midwifery in the UK and the review and synthesis of the results of randomized controlled trials in midwifery-related areas).

3. An overview of midwifery policies in antenatal and postnatal care (a postal survey of policies on antenatal risk assessment and postnatal care in the community).

Although, as we have seen, the NPEU supported midwives undertaking research throughout the 1980s, the MRI offered a more visible focus for midwives who were contemplating undertaking research, and marks the first funded research programme to be headed up by a midwife researcher.

The move of midwifery education into higher education

Alongside this development in midwife-led research, the phrase 'research-based practice' could be heard increasingly frequently as more and more practising midwives began to study research in the context of core research awareness modules. Some went on to undertake research themselves – often within first degree or Master's programmes. The following sentence taken from the preface of a leading midwifery text exemplifies the magnitude of this achievement within just one generation: 'No bibliographic references have been given because of the vast number of sources which have been tapped in compiling the text and because pupil midwives become confused when they study from more than one or two textbooks' (Myles 1952).

Whilst the upsurge of interest in research apparently coincided with the transfer of nursing and midwifery education into higher education (HE) in the early 1990s, it is important to recognize that it actually *predated* the move. However, traditional HE culture has fairly rapidly ensured that research dissertations (whether empirical or based on a literature review) have become firmly embedded in most midwifery degree programmes and teaching staff are now increasingly expected to undertake research as part of their professional activities. The Research Assessment Exercise within the Higher Education sector emphasizes the importance of research activity for all those teaching within HE. Meanwhile, for those working within the clinical field, the *Report of the Taskforce on the Strategy for Research in Nursing, Midwifery and Health Visiting* (Department of Health 1993b) identified the need to enhance the research skills of nurses and midwives in order to facilitate more and better quality research.

The first doctorates awarded to midwives

Midwives were first awarded PhDs during the 1980s, providing a small nucleus of individuals who could embark on postdoctoral research, begin to supervise the research of other midwives and establish research programmes of their own. The award of the first doctorates to midwives is particularly important because, prior to this, all doctoral research had been supervised by academics who were not themselves midwives. Mary Renfrew (then Houston) was the first midwife in the UK to receive a doctorate in 1982 in Edinburgh for a thesis entitled 'Requirements for successful breastfeeding'. Her doctoral research was jointly supervised by the Medical Research Council and the University of Edinburgh. Her three supervisors were Lisbeth Hockey (the well-known nurse researcher), an obstetrician and a biochemist/endocrinologist. However, by the end of 1998 (some 16 years later), it is estimated that there are still fewer than 15 midwives with a doctorate in the UK. Although this number is likely to increase steadily over the coming decade as more and more midwives enrol on Master's and doctoral programmes, it still represents a very small proportion of the 32 700 midwives who have registered their intention to practise with the United Kingdom Central Council for Nursing, Midwifery and Health Visiting (UKCC).

Entries in the Midwifery Research Database (MIRIAD) enable us to chart the steady growth in research undertaken by midwives, with only one study recorded with a start date before 1975, and after that the recorded start dates are as follows:

1976 – 1980	21
1981 – 1985	41
1986 – 1990	117
1991 – 1995	192.

(These data were extracted from McCormick & Renfrew 1997.)

Given this steady upward trend, with a near doubling of the number of studies every five years, it is highly likely that the next five-year period (1996–2000) will continue to reflect an increase in the volume of research in midwifery. The midwife-led research undertaken during the past two decades demonstrates a clear link with practice: the majority (75%) of the 393 studies recorded on MIRIAD had a clinical focus (306), with 23% having a management focus (91), 18% an educational focus (69), and just 1% were categorized as historical (4). Studies with more than one focus have been included in more than one of these categories (data extracted from McCormick & Renfrew 1996, 1997, 1998).

THE EMERGING PLURALISM OF RESEARCH IN MIDWIFERY

A reader of health care research literature might be forgiven for becoming irritated by what Oakley (1998) refers to as 'paradigm disputes and boundary marking'. The contribution of the randomized controlled trial, in particular, continues to be debated (see, for example, Bond 1991, Black 1994, Hicks 1998, Shuldham & Hiley 1997). Against such a background, Sackett & Wennberg (1997) offer some sound advice:

'The argument is not about the inherent value of the different approaches and the worthiness of the investigators who use them. The issue is which way of answering the specific question before us provides the most valid, useful answer. Health and health care would be better served if investigators redirected the energy they currently spend bashing the research approaches they don't use into increasing the validity, power, and productivity of the ones they do.'

The special relationship and close contact midwives have with women throughout pregnancy and birth places them in a unique position to identify a range of issues and research questions that are important to mothers and their families. Indeed, this point was made by Iain Chalmers to members of the Health Committee, who were preparing the second report of the maternity services, during a visit to the NPEU: 'he felt midwives "ask different questions" and that such research is likely to be of benefit to future maternity care. We are persuaded that midwives have much to contribute to research' (House of Commons Health Committee 1992). Midwives tend to use a broader range of research methodologies to tackle these 'different questions' than do their medical colleagues.

The contribution of different research perspectives

There is a clear need for randomized controlled trials (RCTs) to investigate cause and effect relationships and the effectiveness of specific interventions in midwifery care. This not only includes innovations and new practices, but also – and this is far more threatening – activities that are well-established and routinely implemented; what Baker (1998) refers to as the 'sacred cows'. An example of one such recent trial, funded by the Department of Health, investigated the care of the perineum during the second stage of labour (McCandlish et al 1998). In this trial, 5471 eligible women were randomly allocated to either the 'hands on' method in which midwives use their hands to put pressure on the baby's head and 'guard' the perineum, or the 'hands poised' method where the midwife does not touch the baby's head or the woman's perineum, allowing spontaneous delivery of the shoulders. This study, led by a midwife and published in the *British Journal of Obstetrics and Gynaecology* in December 1998, was selected by the editor as 'an example of how a randomized trial should be reported: detailed descriptions of the primary hypothesis being tested; an estimation of the number of women required based upon this hypothesis; the method of randomization and concealment of the allocation until the point of treatment; and the training of the midwives in the two forms of treatment. Thus readers can be reassured that the study is valid and that bias has been minimized' (Grant 1998).

RCTs do not, however, allow midwives and social scientists to address the full health care research agenda. Important questions relating to women's perceptions and experiences of pregnancy and childbirth are not amenable to study through any form of experimental research. So, alongside positivist research, and equally important, have been studies designed to explore different aspects of women's perceptions and experiences in all their richness and diversity. Those working in the maternity services need to know more about what it feels like to be pregnant, to have a baby in the special care baby unit, to lose a baby, and so on. In order to explore areas such as these, researchers need to work within the naturalistic perspective (paradigm) and employ research methodologies such as ethnography, phenomenology and grounded theory.

An analysis of methodology

The studies recorded in MIRIAD demonstrate that many more RCTs have been undertaken by midwives than by nurses; indeed, the need for nurses to become more involved in RCTs has been argued by Cullum (1998). Of the 276 structured abstracts included in MIRIAD up until the beginning of February 1998, 43 (or 16%) were RCTs and a further 9 were case control studies. Trials such as these enable midwives to investigate the effectiveness of specific aspects of care and to make an important contribution to the current drive towards evidence-based health care within the maternity services through the development of systematic reviews and national clinical guidelines.

Perhaps not surprisingly, survey research continues to be the most popular research methodology (144 studies, or 52%), followed by experimental research including RCTs (52 studies, 19%), case study research (24 studies, 9%), ethnography (22 studies, 8%), action research (13 studies) and historical research (7 studies). A further 56 studies were recorded as 'other category', but, on closer examination, several of these were described as phenomenological and a few involved grounded theory. Midwives have, therefore, moved beyond the quantitative research versus qualitative research debate to value different forms of knowledge derived from different types of research. This will certainly strengthen the future of the midwifery profession by ensuring that practice is underpinned by insights derived from different research traditions. Midwives have begun to address what Wilson-Barnett (1998) refers to as the 'intellectual challenge to understanding the different types of research approaches and the evidence they provide for practice'.

The distinctiveness of naturalistic methodologies

Ethnography

Ethnography, with its roots in anthropology, appears to be the naturalistic methodology most widely used by midwives. It is concerned with studying people's behaviour as part of their environment, based on the assumption that we cannot make sense of people's actions without observing them in context. The aim is to understand a person's way of life from the viewpoint of the participants themselves. The focus is on individuals, not in isolation, but in relation to their organizations, communities, customs and culture. Hunt's ethnographic study of a labour ward is perhaps one of the best-known early studies undertaken by a midwife. As Hunt & Symonds (1995) argue, 'It is only by examining a culture in all its richness, intensity, colour, taste and volume that new facets of midwifery can be uncovered, described and given serious thought and consideration'.

Phenomenology

Phenomenology (associated primarily with philosophy and the work of Husserl and Heidegger), on the other hand, seeks to understand an individual's lived experience of a phenomenon such as being pregnant or breastfeeding. The aim is to develop insights which provide a detailed picture of the phenomenon in question from the perspective of those involved. This is achieved by allowing those participating in the study to describe how they experience a particular aspect of their lives.

Grounded theory

Grounded theory differs from ethnography and phenomenology in that its main purpose is to *explain* rather than to *describe* phenomena. Developed in the 1960s by two sociologists, grounded theory aims to generate explanatory theory from the data that are gathered. According to McFarlane (1977), it is an important methodology for practice disciplines such as midwifery and nursing. Using a grounded theory approach, Barclay and Rogan and their colleagues developed a theory about the experience of motherhood and becoming a mother (Barclay et al 1997, Rogan et al 1997). Grounded theory helps us to challenge received wisdom about everyday experiences and events.

Achieving greater clarity in research in midwifery

As midwives and other health services researchers embrace this broad range of research methodologies drawn from both positivist and naturalistic perspectives, it is clearly important to acknowledge their distinctiveness. It should not be acceptable simply to categorize a research study as being either 'qualitative' or 'quantitative' (or even both!). Such terms should only be used to describe the *type of data* that are generated – quantitative (numerical) data or qualitative (descriptive or narrative) data. Since a specific methodology can generate both quantitative and qualitative data, it is inappropriate to refer to the methodology itself as being either quantitative or qualitative. These terms nevertheless continue to be used in the nursing and midwifery research literature and only serve to confuse.

There is also the danger that inexperienced researchers fail to differentiate between the various research methodologies within the naturalistic perspective. Using the example of grounded theory and phenomenology, Baker, Wuest & Stem (1992) warn of the dangers of what they term 'method slurring', which occurs when researchers select aspects from different methodologies and combine them within their own study. When this is done, the resultant research may be savagely critiqued, thereby rendering the results of the study questionable and wasting valuable time and resources invested in the study. Some of the entries in MIRIAD are confusing because terms such as 'qualitative/quantitative', 'simple descriptive study' and 'descriptive qualitative' are used to describe the research design. A handful of studies were recorded as 'ethnography/ phenomenology' or as 'ethnography/grounded theory'. This suggests that there continues to be some confusion surrounding methodological issues, particularly in relation to different types of naturalistic research. (It is important to bear in mind that the studies entered on MIRIAD have not been subject to peer review and the information is provided by the researchers themselves.)

Furthermore, some researchers fail to distinguish between the *research methodology* (e.g. RCT, survey, ethnography) and the *research methods* used to collect and analyse data (such as a questionnaire, a semi-structured interview, or a rating scale). A brief look at the structured abstracts of the research papers published in all four issues of the journal, *Midwifery*, in 1998 suggests that, whilst the majority of survey and experimental studies are appropriately described, there is sometimes a lack of clarity with regard to naturalistic research. Some researchers label the design of their study mainly in terms of a general descriptor and the data collection method rather than the methodology (e.g. 'data were collected by postal questionnaire'; 'qualitative research using in-depth, semi-structured interviews'; 'an ethnographic interview and participant observation with women ...'; 'a descriptive study using screening questionnaires and semi-structured interviews'; 'an in-depth qualitative study of 37 women'). Others use the descriptor 'a qualitative study' and then add 'using a phenomenological approach' to highlight the methodology, or 'qualitative using grounded theory'. It should, however, be noted that papers published in recent nursing and medical journals highlight similar issues in relation to naturalistic methodologies, reflecting perhaps the relative newness of these approaches within health care research more generally.

These and other related issues highlight the need for good supervision. If a midwife cannot be supervised by an experienced researcher who combines a knowledge of midwifery with a good track record of using a particular methodology, then it is important to seek out two supervisors who between them have the necessary skills. If this is not possible, then it is really important for midwives to seek methodological expertise to ensure the study is well designed and that appropriate guidance is available at every stage of data collection and analysis. Sound research education and training is essential if midwives are either to lead or to contribute as equals to multi-disciplinary research and, following the implementation of the *Culyer Report* (Department of Health 1994) discussed in Chapter 3, to compete successfully for research funds.

Information about funding for the 29 new studies entered onto MIRIAD during 1997 and the 20 studies in 1998 demonstrates that midwives have been able to attract financial support for research from a range of sources including the Department of Health/Scottish Office, regional health authorities/NHS Executive, health authorities, NHS trusts, the English National Board for Nursing, Midwifery and Health Visiting, the European Union (small grants), charitable trusts, the Health Education Authority and various commercial companies (McCormick & Renfrew, 1997, 1998). Many of these grants will only have been awarded following extensive peer review, demonstrating that a few midwives are already competing successfully in the increasingly competitive world of research. Robust research training schemes are vital for midwives (and nurses) if they are to take advantage of the extensive R&D funding currently available (see Chapter 3) and in order to ensure that midwives contribute to, and sometimes lead, multi-disciplinary health services research in the future.

The underlying epistemology of the different research approaches means that different procedures are needed to ensure rigour and different criteria should be used to evaluate the research. Research undertaken within the positivist perspective usually aims, through careful sampling procedures, to be generalizable. Rigour is achieved by testing the reliability and validity of the various techniques and measurement tools used to gather data. Within the naturalistic tradition, however, research is evaluated through an audit trail and judgements are made about the extent to which all the steps taken in the process of collecting and analysing the data are traceable. Whilst such accounts are context-specific and the findings cannot be generalized or tell us about the effectiveness of specific outcomes, the insights derived can provide midwives with an important 'mirror' which helps them to reflect on their own practice.

It should be apparent from this brief overview that, in spite of its relatively brief history, research in midwifery is beginning to reflect true methodological pluralism, enabling researchers to tackle the range of issues that those working within the maternity services need to understand in order to deliver quality care. This highlights that although evidence generated by RCTs dominates in medicine, a far broader understanding of what counts as evidence is needed in midwifery. Whilst there is already a well-developed methodology to synthesize the evidence from RCTs within a systematic review, further work is required on how best to synthesize the insights derived from research undertaken within the naturalistic perspective which is context-specific (Noblit & Hare 1988). Sandelowski et al (1997) coin the term 'metasynthesis' to describe the complex process of 'carefully peeling away the surface layers of studies to find their hearts and souls in a way that does least damage to them'. They stress the importance of preserving the integrity of each study and acknowledge the difficulties associated with deciding whether individual studies address the same substantive phenomenon, event or experience.

Lay perspectives in research in midwifery

With the current political focus on consumer involvement in all aspects of health care, it is hardly surprising that this includes research. This has also coincided with a mandate from the NHS R&D strategy to shift from research that is predominantly investigator-led (where the focus of the research is largely determined by the particular interests of those carrying out the research and local need) towards problem-led research (Department of Health, 1993c), thereby opening up the debate about who should be involved in setting the research agenda and identifying research priorities. Perinatal research has led the way in actively involving women and user groups in various aspects of research.

In maternity care, the 'lay perspective' includes women and organizations such as the National Childbirth Trust (NCT) that represent the interests of pregnant women, mothers and their babies. According to Entwistle et al (1998), lay involvement may be beneficial at a number of different points during the research process. Lay contribution may influence: (a) the drawing up of research priorities and identification of important research problems/questions; (b) the design of a study and the way in which it is executed, including commenting on protocols, preparing information for research participants and possibly recruiting participants; and (c) the interpretation of research findings and their effective dissemination and implementation.

Although this topic is discussed more fully in Chapter 5, one study will be mentioned briefly here to highlight the contribution that midwives have made to the wider debate. In a multi-centre, randomized controlled trial to investigate the effectiveness of treatments for women with inverted and flat (non-protractile) nipples (referred to as the MAIN trial), the research question was generated by members of the NCT and by midwives. The study was designed to involve practising midwives and NCT members as active collaborators, which included the important task of recruiting participants to the four arms of the trial. Whilst such an approach goes some way towards operationalizing the vision of the way in which women could become more involved in planning and conducting research that is truly 'with women' rather than 'on women', it also highlighted a number of practical problems including communication difficulties, levels of support from midwifery managers, lack of time, and overwork resulting in tiredness (see Renfrew and McCandlish 1992 for a fuller discussion). This study serves as a reminder of some of the major challenges associated with involving midwives and volunteer mothers in the organization of any large-scale research study.

THE WAY AHEAD

The importance of all midwives being research aware within an evidence-based culture has already been argued. Alongside research awareness, we need more and more midwives to undertake research training programmes that will enable individual researchers to develop methodological expertise. In the longer term, we need experienced researchers to come together to create research programmes with a particular focus. Such centres of excellence should then contribute to the future evidence base of maternity care and also provide an ideal environment within which to train a future generation of researchers. As we have seen, the NPEU has offered such an environment since the 1980s and, more recently, so has the Mother and Infant Research Unit at the University of Leeds. The latter is staffed, in 1998, by an experienced multi-disciplinary research group comprised of four midwives, a sociologist (who is also a midwife), a research psychologist, and a physiologist who has focused on physiological and clinical research into breastfeeding. The unit's research programme:

- 'is multi-disciplinary and uses a wide range of research methods
- has close collaborative links with individuals and organizations locally, regionally, nationally and internationally
- is informed by the views of service users and practitioners
- is informed by, and works to inform, the priorities of relevant bodies including funding agencies' (Mother and Infant Research Unit, *First Report* 1994 1997).

Within this programme there are core themes (horizontal themes) and key topics (vertical themes). The two current key topics are breastfeeding and women's well-being after birth. The core themes are the organization of maternity services (including primary care and the role and work of caregivers); the well-being of childbearing women; reducing inequalities in health and in the delivery of care; the involvement of consumers in research (including the assessment of the views of those participating in research); the development of appropriate research methods; and the dissemination and implementation of research findings and evidence-based practice.

There are currently three PhD students attached to this programme (a midwife, a chemist and a psychologist, funded by Trent Region, the Ministry of Agriculture, Fisheries and Food, and the Medical Research

Council respectively). Here, then, we see how inter-disciplinary collaboration has led, within a relatively short time-span of 3 years, to the development of a thriving research programme that has already resulted in five funded studies and commissioned projects that have been completed, and nine funded studies that are ongoing.

Research in midwifery has clearly come a long way since 1975, but there is still plenty of scope to develop research capacity further and thereby enhance the evidence base of maternity care. More midwives need to acquire research skills. Linked to this is the need for more centres of excellence such as the NPEU and the Mother and Infant Research Unit, and for research programmes that can offer support to both novice researchers and postgraduate students. This should result in a growing research community and culture in midwifery where the pursuit of scholarship can flourish. Progress should also be reflected in higher scores in the Research Assessment Exercise (RAE) – an indicator of the quality and volume of research output of UK academic departments. This score determines the amount of research funding the host institution is awarded from the Higher Education Funding Councils (see Chapter 3).

In this chapter we have seen that much of the research to which midwives contribute is multi-disciplinary. In the early years this may have been largely a pragmatic means of acquiring research training and supervision, rather than a reflection of a commitment to a multi-disciplinary ideology. Since then there has been a general move towards collaborative health care research within the health services, with uni-disciplinary research increasingly regarded as being inward-looking and unduly protective. However, the *Report of the Taskforce for Research in Nursing, Midwifery and Health Visiting* (Department of Health 1993b) argued for ring-fenced funding to enable nurses, midwives and health visitors to 'catch up' with their other health care colleagues. In order to try to differentiate between the rhetoric and the reality of multi-disciplinary research it will be important to see how often midwives lead collaborative research projects (as Renfrew and Smith argue they should in Chapter 3), rather than always being cast as junior partners in relation to medical colleagues, psychologists, sociologists and so on. Only then will true collegiality among health professionals have been achieved in the context of research.

But where is the policy that is guiding research in midwifery? The Centre for Policy in Nursing Research – a joint initiative between the London School of Hygiene and Tropical Medicine and the Royal College of Nursing (and funded for five years by the Nuffield Provincial Hospitals Trust) – has been established in response to specific recommendations in the *Report of the Taskforce for Research in Nursing, Midwifery and Health Visiting* (Department of Health 1993b). The remit of this centre is to develop policies for research in nursing in the future following an audit of current levels of research activity. Whilst it remains to be seen what will emerge from this centre, it does raise the question of where policy for research in midwifery is created and whether it is simply enough to leave it up to those individuals who have so far been successful in attracting research funding and who are beginning to establish research programmes and units.

Conclusion

In 1992, Luker (then Professor of Community Nursing at the University of Liverpool) commented on the 'growing recognition of the scientific merit and high quality of much nursing research.' Certainly, the same could be said of research in midwifery in 1998. The future offers many exciting opportunities as midwives, along with other health care professionals, embrace the challenging research agenda of providing a sound research basis to support evidence-based practice. The commitment and contribution of midwives is growing and there is every reason to believe that this will continue to develop apace. This chapter testifies to the diversity of research in midwifery.

As we approach the millennium midwives should be justifiably proud of their research tradition which has always reflected the needs of women. To provide midwifery care that is both effective and sensitive to the concerns of women and their families, midwives must continue to nurture the relationship between practice and research by contributing to the health care research agenda.

FURTHER READING

Baker M, Kirk S *Research and Development for the NHS: evidence, evaluation and effectiveness*, 2nd edn Oxford: Radcliffe Medical Press; 1998
  An excellent overview of the new NHS Research and Development Programme.
Bowling A *Research Methods in Health: investigating health and health services* Buckingham: Open University Press; 1997
  This text offers an accessible introduction to research methods including a chapter on research paradigms and describing the philosophical underpinnings of different types of research.
Crotty M *The Foundations of Social Research: meaning and perspective in the research process* London: Sage; 1998
  In this text, Crotty examines the epistemological origins of positivism, constructionism, interpretivism, critical theory, feminism and postmodernism. This is highly recommended for students and researchers who are interested in the links between philosophy and research methodology in the social and health sciences.
Traynor M, Rafferty AM, *The NHS R&D Context for Nursing Research: a working paper* London: Centre for Policy in Nursing Research; 1997
  Although written from a nursing perspective, this important report outlines the early work undertaken by the Centre for Policy in Nursing Research. It provides a summary of recent policy initiatives and highlights the complex factors that can promote or inhibit the successful development of research in the health services context.
Smith P *Nursing research: setting new agendas* London: Arnold; 1998
  Whilst the focus of this edited collection is mainly nursing, it explores some key issues

that are equally important for midwives and health visitors, including ways of taking the research agenda forward into the next century.

REFERENCES

Baker MR 'Challenging Ignorance' in Baker M, Kirk S, *Research and Development for the NHS: evidence, evaluation and effectiveness*, 2nd edn. Oxford: Radcliffe Medical Press; 1998

Baker C, Wuest J, Stern PN 'Method Slurring: the grounded theory/phenomenology example' *Journal of Advanced Nursing* 1992; **17(11):** 1355–1360

Barclay L, Everitt L, Rogan F, Schmied V, Wyllie A 'Becoming a Mother – an analysis of women's experience of early motherhood' *Journal of Advanced Nursing* 1997; **25(4):** 719–728

Black N 'Why We Need Qualitative Research' *Journal of Epidemiology and Community Health* 1994; **48:** 425–426

Bond S 'Experimental Research in Nursing: necessary but not sufficient' in Kitson A *Nursing: art and science* London: Chapman and Hall; 1991

Cartwright A *The Dignity of Labour: a study of childbearing and induction* London: Tavistock; 1979

Chalmers I 'Evaluating the Effects of Care During Pregnancy and Childbirth' in Chalmers I, Enkin M, Keirse MJNC *Effective Care in Pregnancy and Childbirth* Volumes 1 and 2 Oxford: Oxford University Press; 1989

Chalmers I, Enkin M, Keirse MJNC *Effective Care in Pregnancy and Childbirth* Volumes 1 and 2 Oxford: Oxford University Press; 1989

Cullum N 'Clinical Effectiveness in Nursing' *NT Research* 1998; **3(1):** 15–18

Department of Health *Research for Health: a research and development strategy for the NHS* London: HMSO; 1991

Department of Health *Changing Childbirth* Part 1: Report of the Expert Maternity Group London: HMSO; 1993a

Department of Health *Report of the Taskforce on the Strategy for Research in Nursing, Midwifery and Health Visiting* London: HMSO; 1993b

Department of Health *Research for Health* London: Department of Health; 1993c

Department of Health *Supporting Research and Development in the NHS* (Chairman: Professor Anthony Culyer) London: HMSO; 1994

Department of Health and Social Security *Report of the Committee on Nursing* (Chairman: Asa Briggs) London: HMSO; 1972

Entwistle VA, Renfrew MJ, Yearley S, Forrester J, Lamont T 'Lay Perspectives: advantages for health research' *British Medical Journal* 1998; **316(7):** 463–466

Garcia J, Garforth S, Ayers S 'The Policy and Practice in Midwifery Study: introduction and methods' *Midwifery* 1987; **3(1):** 2–9

Garcia J, Garforth S 'Labour and Delivery Routines in English Consultant Maternity Units' *Midwifery* 1989; **5(4):** 155–162

Garforth S, Garcia J 'Admitting – a weakness or a strength? Routine admission of a woman in labour' *Midwifery* 1987; **3(2):** 10–24

Garforth S, Garcia J 'breastfeeding Policies in Practice – no wonder they get confused' *Midwifery* 1989; **5(2):** 75–83

Grant J 'Editor's choice' *British Journal of Obstetrics and Gynaecology* 1998; **105:** vii

Grant A, Sleep J, Ashurst H, Spencer JAD 'Dyspareunia Associated with the Use of Glycerol-impregnated Catgut to Repair Perineal Trauma – report of a three-year follow-up study' *British Journal of Obstetrics and Gynaecology* 1989a; **96:** 741–743

Grant A, Sleep J, McIntosh J, Ashurst H 'Ultrasound and Pulsed Electromagnetic Energy Treatment for Perineal Trauma: a randomized placebo-controlled trial' *British Journal of Obstetrics and Gynaecology* 1989b; **96:** 434–439

Hicks C 'The Randomized Controlled Trial: a critique' *Nurse Researcher* 1998; **6(1):** 19–32

House of Commons Health Committee *Second Report on the Maternity Services* Volume 1 (Chairman: Lord Winterton) London: HMSO; 1992

Hunt S, Symonds A *The Social Meaning of Midwifery* Basingstoke: Macmillan; 1995

Kitzinger S *Giving Birth: the parents' emotions in childbirth* London: Gollancz; 1971

Kitzinger S *Some Mothers' Experiences of Induced Labour* London: National Childbirth Trust; 1975

Kitzinger S *The Experience of Breastfeeding* Harmondsworth: Penguin; 1979

Luker K 'Research and Development in Nursing' *Journal of Advanced Nursing* 1992; **17(10):** 1151–1152

Macfarlane A, Mugford M *Birth Counts: statistics of pregnancy and childbirth*, London: HMSO; 1984

Macfarlane A, Mugford M, Johnson A, Garcia J *Counting the Changes in Childbirth: trends and gaps in national statistics*, Oxford: National Perinatal Epidemiology Unit; 1995

McCandlish R, Bowler U, van Asten H, Berridge G, Winter C, Sames C, Garcia J, Renfrew M, Elbourne D 'A Randomized Controlled Trial of the Perineum During the Second Stage of Normal Labour' *British Journal of Obstetrics and Gynaecology* 1998; **105:** 1262–1272

McCormick F, Renfrew MJ *The Midwifery Research Database MIRIAD: A sourcebook of information about research in midwifery* Second edition Hale, Cheshire: Books for Midwives Press; 1996

McCormick F, Renfrew MJ *The Midwifery Research Database MIRIAD: A sourcebook of information about research in midwifery* Third edition Hale, Cheshire: Books for Midwives Press; 1997

McCormick F, Renfrew MJ *The Midwifery Research Database MIRIAD: A register of information about research in midwifery,* Hale, Cheshire: Books for Midwives Press; 1998

McFarlane JK *The Proper Study of the Nurse: an account of the first two years of a research project 'The study of nursing care', including a study of relevant background literature* London: Royal College of Nursing; 1970

McFarlane JK 'Developing a Theory of Nursing: the relation of theory to practice, education and research' *Journal of Advanced Nursing* 1977; **2(3):** 261–270

Mother and Infant Research Unit *First Report 1994–1997* Leeds: University of Leeds; 1998

Myles M, *Myles' Textbook for Midwives* Edinburgh: Churchill Livingstone; 1952

National Perinatal Epidemiology Unit *National Perinatal Epidemiology Unit Report 1989 and 1990* Oxford: NPEU; 1991

National Perinatal Epidemiology Unit *National Perinatal Epidemiology Unit Report 1993* Oxford: NPEU; 1994

Noblit GW, Hare RD *Meta-ethnography: synthesising qualitative studies* Newbury Park, California: Sage; 1988

Oakley A *From Here to Eternity: becoming a mother* Harmondsworth: Penguin; 1979

Oakley A *Women Confined: towards a sociology of childbirth* Oxford: Martin Robertson; 1980

Oakley A 'Living in Two Worlds' *British Medical Journal* 1998; **316:** 482–483

Peckham M 'Preliminary statement' in Department of Health *Research For Health: a research and development strategy for the NHS*, London: HMSO; 1991

Proud J, Grant AM 'Third Trimester Placental Grading by Ultrasonography as a Test of Fetal Wellbeing' *British Medical Journal* 1987; **294:** 1641–1644

Renfrew MJ, McCandlish R 'With Women: new steps in research in midwifery', in Roberts H *Women's Health Matters* London: Routledge; 1992

Rogan F, Schmied V, Barclay L, Wyllie A 'Becoming a Mother – developing a new theory of early childhood' *Journal of Advanced Nursing* 1997; **25(5):** 877–885

Romney ML 'Predelivery Shaving: an unjustified assault?' *Journal of Obstetrics and Gynaecology* 1980; **1:** 33–35

Romney ML, Gordon H 'Is Your Enema Really Necessary?' *British Medical Journal* 1981; **282:** 1269–1271

Sackett DL, Wennberg JE 'Choosing the Best Research Design for Each Question' *British Medical Journal* 1997; **315:** 1636

Sandelowski M, Docherty S, Emden C 'Qualitative Metasynthesis: issues and techniques' *Research in Nursing and Health* 1997; **20(4):** 365–371

Shuldham C, Hiley C 'Randomized Controlled Trials in Clinical Practice: the continuing debate' *NT Research* 1997; **2(2):** 128–134

Sleep J 'Episiotomy in Normal Delivery' *Nursing Times* 1984a; **80(47):** 28–30

Sleep J 'Management of the Perineum' *Nursing Times* 1984b; **80(48):** 51–54

Sleep J, Grant A, Garcia J, Elbourne D, Spencer J, Chalmers I 'West Berkshire Perineal Management Trial' *British Medical Journal* 1984; **289:** 587–590

Sleep J 'Things I wished I'd known before I started' *Midwifery* 1985; **1(1):** 54–57

Sleep J 'Perineal Care: a series of five randomized controlled trials', in Robinson S, Thomson AM *Midwives, Research and Childbirth* Volume 2 London: Chapman and Hall; 1991

Sleep J, Grant A 'Pelvic Floor Exercises in Postnatal Care' *Midwifery* 1987a; **3:** 158–164

Sleep J, Grant A 'West Berkshire Perineal Management Trial: three year follow-up' *British Medical Journal* 1987b; **295:** 749–751

Sleep J, Grant A 'Effects of Salt and Savlon Bath Concentrate Post-partum' *Nursing Times* 1988; **84(21):** 55–57

Spencer J, Grant A, Elbourne D, Garcia J, Sleep J, 'A Randomized Controlled Comparison of Glycerol-impregnated Catgut with Untreated Chromic Catgut for the Repair of Perineal Trauma' *British Journal of Obstetrics and Gynaecology* 1986; **93:** 426–430

Standing Maternity and Midwifery Advisory Committee *Report on Domiciliary Midwifery and Maternity Bed Needs* (The Peel Report) London: HMSO; 1970

Tew M 'The Case Against Hospital Deliveries: the statistical evidence', in Kitzinger S, Davis JA *The Place of Birth: a study of the environment in which birth takes place with special reference to home confinements* Oxford: Oxford University Press; 1978

Tew M 'The Safest Place of Birth: further evidence' *The Lancet* 1979; **i:** 1388–1390

The Lancet 'Servicing Perinatal Research' *The Lancet* 1991; **338:** 1564

Wilson-Barnett J 'Evidence for Nursing Practice – an overview' *NT Research* 1998; **3(1):** 12–14

Young D 'Some Thoughts on Collaboration in Perinatal Research' *Birth* 1991; **18(3):** 135–136

3

Research and development in the NHS

Mary Renfrew and Michael Smith

KEY ISSUES

- Evolution of the NHS Research and Development (R&D) strategy
- Definitions and terminology of R&D
  - *Research or development?*
  - *Biomedical research and Health Services Research (HSR)*
  - *Implicit and explicit research*
  - *Multi-disciplinary research*
- Evidence-based practice
  - *Deriving evidence*
  - *Who is the evidence for?*
  - *Evidence into practice*
- Research quality
  - *Source of funding*
  - *External peer review*
  - *Publication of research findings*
- Research funding
  - *Response mode*
  - *Identified priorities – Health Technology Assessment*
  - *Priority setting for research in the NHS*
  - *The Culyer initiative*
- Guidance for health care professionals undertaking research in the NHS.

INTRODUCTION

With the celebration in 1998 of the 50th anniversary of the formation of the NHS, it is almost inconceivable to consider that for over 40 years there was no coherent strategy for research and development, or R&D. It would be taken for granted in any medium sized or large company, let alone in an organization the size of the NHS, that R&D would play a key role in any future success. In 1998/9 the NHS had a budget of £423 million for research. In addition, a significant proportion of other organizations' funding is spent within the NHS; the total budget of the medical research charities was £340 million in 1995/6 and the Medical Research Council (MRC) spend was £282 million in 1996/7.

When planning for R&D in the NHS started in the early 1990s, we might have been advised 'if you want to go there, you shouldn't start from here'. A challenge evolved, not only to identify, instigate and fund new policies, but also to undo and refocus policies and attitudes that had developed over the years. Some activities were considered erroneously as R&D, and in other cases the disagreements about R&D policy were a consequence of the varying perceptions of different professional groups, all of whom had differing interpretations about the meaning, definition and importance of R&D.

Prior to the 1990s, though there had been no R&D *policy*, there had always been considerable research and development in the NHS. Generally it was uncoordinated. It was simply accepted that medical and scientific staff undertook R&D as part of their employment. Often, however, there was no consideration given to the relationship between R&D and subsequent changes in practice. In addition, there was little or no recognition of the role and potential contribution of other groups such as midwives, nurses and therapists. It had been recognized that the larger hospitals, often attached to medical schools, were more expensive to run than smaller District General Hospitals and, as a consequence, they received additional funding via SIFTR (service increment for teaching and research). Though there was considerable funding in the health service, which fell under this heading, there was no explicit relationship between the research monies falling under the 'R' component of SIFTR and the actual R&D activity within the NHS. Considerable research was also funded by research councils and charitable research funding bodies, much of it high quality, and it was assumed that the NHS would support and provide resources for such activity to take place. Similarly, commercial companies undertook clinical trials within the NHS and supported the resources used to a greater or lesser degree.

Research training and education was patchy in some specialist areas and non-existent in others; indeed, in areas where junior staff undertook research, there was little or no formal training. It seemed to be assumed that research methodologies and techniques would be learned largely by osmosis. Curiously, it was often considered that research consisted of gaining experience in a particular technique and applying it to a small group of patients, with little or no attention paid to research methodology or critical appraisal.

It was into this anarchic and not particularly cost effective environment that the NHS R&D strategy was launched in the early 1990s. This chapter sets out the evolution of the NHS R&D initiative and highlights key components of R&D in the NHS that are now central for health care and which are increasingly held up as an example by other countries.

EVOLUTION OF THE NHS R&D STRATEGY

The first Director of R&D in the NHS was Professor, now Sir, Michael Peckham, who was appointed in 1991. He was a member of the Management Executive of the NHS, reporting directly to the Chief Executive of the NHS, and was advised by a new committee, the CRDC (Central Research and Development Committee) which was set up to 'to strengthen through the research and development programme the scientific basis for defining strategies in health care, operational policy and management'. The CRDC strategy increased the emphasis on health care and has had considerable implications for the way in which research has traditionally been pursued and funded within teaching hospitals. The membership of the CRDC covers a wide range of specialities from the basic biomedical sciences through to the social sciences and includes a range of different health professionals.

CRDC members were not chosen to represent their particular speciality but to give broad consideration to the whole area of R&D in the NHS. The committee also included, as ex-officio members, the Chief Nurse, the Chief Medical Officer and the Director of the MRC. From the start there was a need for a 'hearts and minds' exercise to achieve a substantial change in attitude, an approach which is still continuing.

It should be remembered that the R&D initiative in the NHS was not an isolated change in the research environment in the United Kingdom. There had been other major changes, which were significant in themselves, as well as ones which impacted on the NHS research environment; these are listed in Table 3.1.

In addition to specific events there were significant evolutionary developments in research culture between the late 1980s and the mid-1990s. The changes were various but interlinked, the common feature being the emphasis on eventual health or patient outcome and also benefits for the NHS. These included:

1. the development of health services research (HSR)
2. the publication of *Effective Care in Pregnancy and Childbirth* which signalled the importance of systematically reviewing and critically appraising existing evidence and resulted in the formation of the Cochrane collaboration
3. growing recognition of the importance of implementing research findings (often referred to as 'development') as indicated by the growth in interest in 'evidence-based medicine or practice'.

A more comprehensive background to the development of the NHS R&D programme, and a critique, has been published (Black 1997).

Since the formation of the CRDC there have been a number of major initiatives in R&D. These include targeted research areas, for example Mother and Child Health, as well as processes for detailed prioritizing and commissioning of research at a national level, such as the Health Technology Assessment programme. The key features are summarized in Table 3.1.

As there was so much to achieve from the start, it was not possible to attempt to find immediate solutions to every aspect of research and development. The targeted research areas such as Mother and Child Health,

Table 3.1 Recent changes in the research environment in the UK

NHS R&D	National Research Environment
1991 Start of the NHS R&D initiative. Appointment of an NHS R&D Director and the creation of the Central Research and Development Committee (CRDC). Publication of 'Research for Health'.	
1992 Publication of Regional R&D plans. UK Cochrane Centre opened in Oxford. Start of nine focused research programmes: (1) asthma management, (2) cardiovascular disease and stroke, (3) cancer, (4) evaluation of methods to promote the implementation of research findings, (5) mental health, (6) mother and child health, (7) physical and complex disabilities, (8) primary/secondary care, (9) primary dental care	Research council dual support system implemented. Funding increasingly associated with grants received rather than block funding given to institutions. Higher Education Funding Council's (HEFC) Research Assessment Exercise (RAE) taken more seriously than previous exercises.
1993 Second version of 'Research for Health' published. DoH taskforce report on research in nursing, midwifery and health visiting. Centre for Reviews and Dissemination opened in York. Start of the Health Technology Assessment Programme.	Polytechnics achieve University status. Increase in expectation of new Universities to become research active. Government White Paper on Science and Technology.
1994 Publication of the 'Culyer' report. CRDC now advises NHS how to invest its R&D funds. Creation of National Forum to bring together the major health-related research funders to provide advice to the NHS.	
1995	Technology Foresight exercise identifies important areas for research in the future, including evidence-based healthcare.
1996 NHS Trusts declare their research activity. Standing advisory group on consumer involvement in NHS R&D.	HEFC Research Assessment Exercise. Colleges of Health become incorporated into Universities.
1997 Trusts submit R&D bids for portfolio or task-linked funding.	RAE rating significantly influences resources to Universities.
1998 NHS Trusts received funding directly associated with research for which they will be accountable. Start of the Service Delivery and Organization Programme. New and Emerging Applications for Technology Programme (subject to ministerial approval).	

having achieved an increase in research activity, have now been replaced by three generic funding streams which cover all clinical areas:

1. Service delivery and organization
2. New and emerging technologies
3. Health Technology Assessment.

Central to the NHS R&D initiative is the support of quality research and the encouragement of research which will improve health care. It is essential that research is not duplicated needlessly and that gaps in knowledge are filled. A description of components of the R&D programme which offer opportunities within midwifery are discussed later in the chapter and full details of the complete programme are available in numerous published reports and on the Internet (NHS R&D website: http://www.open.gov.uk/doh/rdd1.htm)

Definitions and terminology

If you travel in a foreign country, you are likely to get lost unless you know the language. It is helpful, therefore, to explain some of the widely used terminology in order to understand some of the underlying principles which guide the NHS R&D initiative. In some cases, you may find the definitions of terms unfamiliar; it has been our experience that different speciality groups have what amount to different dialects in 'R&D speak'. We hope that the definitions used here can be generally accepted.

Research or development?

The words 'research' and 'development' often seem to go together even though they refer to quite distinct activities which are often pursued separately. *Research* is the activity which seeks to establish new knowledge about a problem or achieve understanding of something which is generalizable and objective. This means that the findings are relevant, and can be applied widely, within the specific area of health care under investigation.

Development, on the other hand, should be considered as the implementation of research findings into specific local circumstances. This may involve additional investigative work and activities to incorporate and implement the appropriate research findings and check local applicability. It is easy to see why R&D are considered together, but the majority of the activity that people view as R&D in fact falls under the development umbrella, as it is concerned with the *implementation* of existing research findings. This in no way diminishes the value of development; indeed it could be argued that the development component of R&D is the more likely to have an impact on service delivery and changes in practice. However, it is essential that such development is founded on good quality research (see Chapter 8).

Biomedical research and health services research (HSR)

Biomedical research investigates the scientific basis of medicine and health; this type of research has been dominant in the past in hospitals. Biomedical research can include the investigation of the biological, molecular and physiological basis of diseases and the human response to disease, as well as the development of new imaging technologies. It involves the scientific investigation of a problem, which, if it yields a solution, may not have an impact on health care in the short term. Though the success rate could be low, results could have major implications for medical and health care.

The Medical Research Council (MRC) definition of *health services research* (HSR) is 'the identification of the health care needs of the community and the study of the provision, effectiveness and use of health services'. It will stress the effect of any procedure or process on the outcome for the patient. Successful HSR should provide results that will lead to a significant improvement to the delivery of health care in the relatively short term. A key feature of the NHS R&D programme is the increased emphasis on HSR as this area of research is likely to have most impact on health care.

Implicit and explicit research

Research can be *implicit* or *explicit*, and this can affect which research problems are investigated and the way in which the research is undertaken. Implicit research describes research determined by the individual researcher or team with no external review. This can result in the following problems and consequences:

- The research undertaken may not be of particularly high priority.
- Many people and places may be pursuing identical research.
- There may be important areas of research that need to be investigated that are not being pursued by anyone.
- Generally there is not good quality assurance of the research.

Explicit research refers to research which responds to external initiatives and priorities. There is a process whereby the project is agreed by others. The move away from implicit and towards explicit research by the CRDC is simply a recognition that there must be a component of research which is targeted to specific needs. It avoids the problems of implicit research and the external refereeing constrains the researcher to consider and implement good quality assurance.

Multi-disciplinary research

A multi-disciplinary philosophy is essential to success in research and has always had a high priority in the NHS R&D initiative. Multi-disciplinary research is fostered and encouraged because it produces better quality and more relevant research findings. The advantages of a multi-disciplinary approach include the pragmatic reason that, within the funding streams of the NHS R&D programme, multi-disciplinary applications have three times the likelihood of success than applications from a single discipline.

We consider the term *multi-disciplinary research* to describe collaboration between different disciplines, each bringing specific expertise and knowledge to the research programme, working together to support the different components. An example of multi-disciplinary research could be a research programme concerned with the cost effectiveness of midwifery services. A team carrying out this programme would require expertise in the area of midwifery, the social sciences, health economics, and experience in data handling, analysis and health informatics. It is essential for all members of the team to be sympathetic to, and have some knowledge of the other components, but also to recognize the high level of expertise which is required in each area if good quality research is to be obtained. Within a multi-disciplinary team, there is a clear need for expertise in research design and methodology, and project management. Such expertise requires training and experience in research, but is not automatically associated with one particular discipline.

Research is often, of course, focused within a specific discipline and it may not *need* to be multi-disciplinary. If this is the case, however, it is important to avoid any sense of separateness or isolation from the mainstream research community. The methodological problems and practical challenges encountered in research in health care are common to all professions working in the field.

Evidence-based practice

Central to research in the NHS in the late 1990s is the philosophy of 'evidence-based medicine', now also known as 'evidence-based practice' (Sackett et al 1997). Experience has shown that this phrase irritates many people who have been engaged in research in medicine and health for many years, because they regard themselves as researchers who have been using evidence throughout their careers. However, given the variations in practice and the availability of different therapies throughout the country, it suggests that the evidence base in health care is often either contradictory, variable or absent (Sackett et al 1996).

Deriving evidence

It is quite useful to consider the three major methods of deriving 'evidence' from research.

1. *Primary research* can be defined as empirical work, which will produce new information from observational or experimental studies.

2. *Secondary research* is analysis of information obtained from primary research, often combining a number of different studies, to extract evidence. Such work should be undertaken using a systematic approach, hence the term 'systematic review'.
3. *Modelling* is the mathematical analysis of available information to interpolate and predict evidence in future changed circumstances.

Within the NHS R&D programme, there has been an emphasis on developing primary research based on the results of secondary research – reviews of existing research. The NHS Centre for Reviews and Dissemination, and the UK Cochrane Centre are both funded by this programme (Renfrew 1997). Systematic reviews are a valuable source of developing and acquiring evidence from a mass of information and the skills learned in systematic reviewing can help researchers design their own primary research to obtain such evidence directly. There is a range of publications which describe this in detail (Antman et al 1992, Oxman & Guyatt 1993, Dickersin et al 1994, Centre for Reviews and Dissemination 1996, Chalmers & Altman 1996).

Who is the evidence for?

We all see problems and have particular expertise in research from our own speciality's perspective, but it is important to remember that the resultant evidence may need to convince individuals from completely different specialities.

At the end of the day, most evidence is for the *benefit of the consumer* – in midwifery, the childbearing woman and her baby. The role and value of the consumer in contributing to research at different stages has, at last, been recognized by the NHS R&D programme. This is a challenging issue, and organizing structures and methods for consumers to contribute positively is not always easy (Entwistle et al 1998; see Chapter 5). The mechanisms for the involvement of consumers and consumer groups are still evolving within the NHS R&D programme.

Evidence into practice

The NHS R&D programme is also funding research into the most effective ways of implementing research evidence in practice, including systematic reviews (co-ordinated by the Cochrane Effective Practice and Organization of Care group (EPOC)) and primary research. A new programme of research on Service Delivery and Organization of Care, similar in scale to the health technology assessment (HTA) programme, was established in 1999. A series of papers on the topic of 'getting research findings into practice' addresses many of the challenges in this field (Haines & Donald

1998, Sheldon et al 1998, Glanville et al 1998, Haynes & Haines 1998, Straus & Sackett 1998, Lilford et al 1998, Bero et al 1998, Garner et al 1998).

Research quality

A key aim within the research community in the UK has been to improve the quality of research. Within the NHS, the relevance of research, that is, the impact on patient outcome, could be regarded as a component of 'quality', but we believe relevance is important enough to be considered separately. In addition to increasing the amount of research that would be perceived as relevant to the needs of the NHS, the actual quality of the research undertaken, in terms of the reliability and applicability of the research output, is also a major factor. When assessing the quality of a research study, a number of factors can be regarded as surrogate indicators of quality. Though they do not guarantee that the research output is of high quality, they are more likely to produce research of high quality.

Source of funding

A number of funding bodies have an extensive peer review process and, therefore, it is likely that any research which is funded would have passed through the appropriate filters to ensure soundness of methodology and appropriate study design. Generally research funded by the research councils, the Wellcome Trust, the National NHS R&D programme and the major charitable funding bodies within the AMRC (Association of Medical Research Charities) falls into this category. Simple receipt of external funding is not necessarily an indication that the research being undertaken is good quality, but the source of the funding is helpful in assessing research quality. Of course funding may not be awarded if the subject is not a high priority for the funding body and so the refusal of funding does not necessarily indicate low quality.

External peer review

The consideration of a research proposal by an individual, or individuals, external to the researcher and with a broad knowledge of research methods and technique is more likely to ensure that the research is of good quality. Remembering the earlier emphasis on multi-disciplinary research, it is generally desirable that external referees should come from a broad range of disciplines and not simply from within a single discipline (see Chapter 13). It follows, therefore, that research applications must not only be carefully written but it must be kept in mind that individuals who are not from your own particular speciality may judge them.

Publication of research findings

It is important to distinguish between academic journals, which concentrate on publishing good quality research output, and professional 'magazines' whose prime purpose is the dissemination of information to the wider body of a particular profession. The two types of publication have quite different mechanisms for considering and accepting articles for publication and the careful refereeing and vetting process undertaken by academic journals is designed specifically to maintain quality. Within a particular field some journals are more highly regarded than others and they may reject a higher proportion of submitted papers allowing them only to publish those of the highest quality.

In the university sector there is a Research Assessment Exercise (RAE) every four to five years. This does not seek to judge the quantity of published research but specifically limits researchers to presenting four papers within a four or five year period, placing a very firm emphasis on quality.

Research funding

There are three main categories of funding:

1. response mode funding
2. funding in response to identified priorities
3. assignment of existing resources within the NHS to specific research activity (the Culyer initiative).

Response mode funding

Up till 5 years ago, the resources within the NHS which funded research could be classified as:

- Funding held at regional level which responded to bids on subjects chosen by the applicants.
- Much greater resources which were tied up in the funding of hospitals and could not be applied to any particular activity that was being undertaken.

This mode of funding is known as *response mode*, where a funding body responds to proposals submitted by researchers who require funds for their own projects. This type of funding has now changed in the NHS. For example, the Regional R&D offices have targeted funding to increase research capacity and training and to promote certain research priorities, decided by them. This is usually in addition to supporting limited responsive mode funding. Regions now fund research fellowships, recognizing the importance of supporting researchers from different constituencies, and specific targeted research training in the areas of health care. It is no longer the case that regional NHS funding is the property of the medical establishment working in the area of biomedical research.

Response mode funding, though now more limited than in the past, still plays an important role for new and established researchers. The policies of many funding bodies differ with regard to the specific details required for a funding application. Some have dedicated funding streams or research fellowships which are earmarked to support new researchers or to provide career development for applicants who wish to focus on research.

Identified priorities – health technology assessment

Of the many new initiatives which invite bids for funding associated with identified priorities, the health technology assessment (HTA) programme is probably the one which offers the most opportunities in the late 1990s. It is one of the main sources of central NHS R&D funding and unlike some others, is an ongoing programme (Smith 1996, HTA website).

The health technology part of HTA is deliberately defined as broadly as possible. It covers any method used by health professionals to promote health, prevent and treat disease and improve rehabilitation and long-term care. It includes the activities of the full range of health care professionals, the use of equipment, practices and procedures and the administration of pharmaceutical products. The assessment component is quite specific. The health technology or practice under assessment should be clearly defined and in sufficiently stable use for it to need assessment. It should be compared with competing health technologies and the effects of no intervention. The end point of the assessment should be improved patient outcome and/or a more cost-effective means of achieving comparable outcomes. It is important to stress that this is *more* than technology evaluation. The HTA programme is not only interested in new technologies and practices, but also existing ones which lack evidence to support their continued use or application.

The programme publishes a brief outline of the current priorities. Short proposals are then invited from any interested researchers: details of the specific research proposed, the multi-disciplinary research team, the specific methodology and study design, the research environment and indications of costings are all requested at this stage. These are considered and successful applicants are invited to submit full proposals which are then evaluated in a further round. The two-stage process is used to minimize the time spent by researchers on preparing unsuccessful full-length proposals.

Priority setting for research in the NHS

The NHS R&D programme has taken steps to set up processes for prioritizing research. Much of this has been done in association with the

HTA programme and successful practices are likely to be used in the other two general funding streams. One of us (MS) is chairman of one of the panels of the HTA programme and an outline is given here of the processes developed by that panel to identify and agree priorities.

Possible priorities are identified each year after an extensive consultation exercise. All are considered by a panel whose membership selection takes account of the following:

- a balance of expertise
- public health and management involvement
- two consumer members
- no vested interests
- an attempt at geographic and gender balance.

In considering the proposed topics, which may amount to several hundred, the following processes are employed:

1. there is no pre-set scoring system and no pre-ranking
2. there is declaration of interests of all panel members when each item is discussed
3. the number of repeated topics is noted
4. output from 'horizon scanning' is noted (this is carried out by a separate panel to identify issues which will be important in the future)
5. consideration is given to previous year's 'near-misses'
6. expert papers are used for detailed clarification
7. output from NHS R&D research and systematic reviews which define research questions is used.

Assigning existing resources: the Culyer initiative

When the NHS R&D strategy was set up, it was recognized that substantial changes could not occur until there was a clear relationship between research activity and research funding within the NHS. This resulted in potentially the most substantial change associated with research in the NHS, known colloquially as the 'Culyer' exercise (Department of Health 1994).

The publication of the *Culyer Report* in 1994 made the following substantial recommendations:

- modify the CRDC and its terms of reference so it has responsibility for the R&D budget
- form a National Forum of R&D funding bodies
- form a single R&D budget with clearly defined sub-streams (NHS R&D, service support etc) and clear and fair principles for competition, contracting and assessment.

These recommendations were introduced into the NHS over a number of years. Several points required substantial effort throughout the NHS, and the exercise played a major role in bringing research onto the agenda of Trust organizations. Intended, and to some extent now realized, consequences of the Culyer exercise at a local level were to improve the quality of NHS R&D, to decrease implicit and to increase explicit R&D, and to provide resources for new R&D. The latter is particularly important for new developments in health care areas.

The implementation of the Culyer process occurred between 1995 and 1998. NHS organizations had to declare the research activity that was being undertaken within their walls with the exception of commercially funded research as it was assumed that this would be completely self-financing. This inventory then had to be related to the amount of NHS resources that they *actually* spent on research, both in terms of supporting externally-funded research and undertaking research within the Trust. During this period of examination NHS organizations experienced no change in funding. They then had to submit a 'Culyer bid' for funding all research across all disciplines within their organization. The bid had to be related to their declaration, if they had submitted one previously.

It was possible for organizations within the NHS to submit Culyer bids even if they had not previously received research funding and, therefore, had not made a declaration. Two types of bid were allowed: a 'portfolio bid' was for large programmes of research and research support over a 3 year period. The second type of funding was 'task linked' bids. These were given for a period of 1 year and institutions were able to submit further task linked bids in later years. Within the Culyer bidding exercise there was no new money to support research. Institutions had to justify receiving the funding they had submitted in their original declaration and make a strong case for any additional money. Increases in funding for some institutions would, as a consequence, result in reduced funding elsewhere.

GUIDANCE FOR MIDWIVES SEEKING FUNDING FROM THE NHS R&D PROGRAMME

In many years of undertaking research in the NHS, we have had to offer advice and guidance to experienced and prospective researchers. The key features of such advice, which could be useful to midwifery researchers, are listed below. We have also given an indication of how the NHS may now be more accommodating of midwives wishing to research.

- *Remember the adage 'don't run before you can walk'.* Funding is increasingly available for bursaries to enable prospective researchers to undertake small projects to gain experience.
- *Recognize that others may not ascribe the same priority to your research topic*

as you do. Increasingly research priorities are defined within the national NHS R&D agenda and locally within 'Culyer' contracts. Accept and take advantage of the opportunities presented by advertised priority areas for research. Study the 'vignettes' that have been prepared by the funders or commissioners, which outline the problems and issues of current interest.

- *Be prepared to shift your research interest; do not remain wedded to the research area of your dissertation or thesis.* Research bids in the NHS increasingly concentrate on the quality of the research environment rather than specific experience in a narrow area.
- *Focus on problem-based research, not speciality-based research.*
- *Consider the outcome and benefits for the patient and NHS, not necessarily what specialists may want.* These two points are now key features of all NHS R&D funding, including local Culyer contracts.
- *Bring together the appropriate multi-disciplinary group, bearing in mind the various audiences for the evidence your research will produce.* This is central to all NHS R&D funding bids. Significant emphasis is placed on the involvement of all relevant health care professionals. Midwives are as capable as anyone else of being leaders of multi-disciplinary research teams.
- *When preparing a grant application, read what the instructions say and follow them.*
- *For quality research seek quality funding.*
- *Remember that grant submissions may not be refereed by experts in your own field.* The two-stage application process often used in the NHS can help to reduce time spent on eventually unsuccessful applications.
- *Use the goodwill, expertise and willingness to give advice of experienced researchers to review research proposals and applications before submission.* The need for improvements in research quality is now recognized at an organizational level and often mentoring systems are set up. Staff can benefit from the expertise of a wide range of mentors.
- *Don't give up.* We cannot pretend that it is easy to do research and that the NHS has removed all the frustrations and potential disappointments. Research will never be easy but opportunities for midwives and other health care professionals are greater now than they have been in the past.

CONCLUSION

Research and development in the NHS has changed dramatically within the 1990s. The key principles of the NHS R&D programme, including prioritizing research topics that matter to the health service, funding quality research, involving a range of perspectives including consumers and linking evidence with practice, are all fundamentally important to research and practice in midwifery. Midwives have been successful in gaining research funds from the R&D programme. It is likely that, as midwives become more experienced in research and more involved in multi-disciplinary research groups, that his success will grow and develop. It is important too that, whenever appropriate, midwives share in the R&D programme by contributing to and working on advisory and priority setting groups.

FURTHER READING

NHS R&D Programme information:
Research and Development: Towards an Evidence-base for Health Services, Public Health and Social Care. Information Packs, Issue 5, March 1988. Available from Department of Health, PO Box 410, Wetherby, LS23 7LN.
NHS Executive 1997 *Research and Development in Primary Care: National Working Group Report.* Available from Department of Health, PO Box 410, Wetherby, LS23 7LN

Useful websites:
MRC: www.mrc.ac.uk
ESRC: www.esrc.ac.uk
Midwifery Research Database (MIRIAD): www.leeds.ac.uk/miru/miriad/home.htm

---

REFERENCES

Antman EM, Lau J, Kupelnick B, Mosteller F, Chalmers TC 'A Comparison of Results of Meta-analyses of Randomized Control Trials and Recommendations of Clinical Experts. Treatments for myocardial infarction' *JAMA* 1992; **268(2):** 240–248
Bero LA, Grilli R, Grimshaw JM, Harvey E, Oxman AD, Thomson MA 'Closing the Gap Between Research and Practice; an overview of systematic reviews of interventions to promote the implementation of research findings' *BMJ* 1998; **317:** 465–468
Black N 'A National Strategy for Research and Development; Lessons from England *Annual Reviews of Public Health* 1997; **18:** 485–505
Centre for Reviews and Dissemination (CRD) 'Undertaking systematic reviews of research on effectiveness *CRD Report 4*; 1996
Chalmers I, Altman D *Systematic Reviews* London: BMJ publishing group; 1996
Department of Health *Supporting Research and Development in the NHS* (the Culyer Report) London: HMSO; 1994
Dickersin K, Scherer R, Lefebvre C 'Identifying Relevant Studies for Systematic Reviews' *BMJ* 1994; **309:** 1286–1291
Entwistle VA, Renfrew MJ, Yearley S, Forrester J, Lamont T 'Lay Perspectives: advantages for health research' *BMJ* 1998; **316:** 463–466
Garner P, Kale R, Dickson R, Dans T, Salinas R 'Implementing Research Findings in Developing Countries' *BMJ* 1998; **317:** 531–535
Glanville J, Haines M, Auston I 'Finding Information on Clinical Effectiveness' *BMJ* 1998; **317:** 200–203
Haines A, Donald A 'Making Better Use of Research Findings' *BMJ* 1998; **317:** 72–75
Haynes B, Haines A 'Barriers and Bridges to Evidence-based Clinical Practice' *BMJ* 1998; **317:** 273–276
Health Technology Assessment website *http://www.soton.ac.uk/~hta/*
Lilford R, Pauker SG, Braunholtz DA, Chard J 'Decision Analysis and the Implementation of Research Findings' *BMJ* 1998; **317:** 405–409
NHS R&D website *http://www.open.gov.uk/doh/rdd1.htm*

Oxman AD, Guyatt GH 'The Science of Reviewing Research' *Ann NY Acad Sci* 1993; **703:** 125–133

Renfrew MJ 'The Development of Evidence-based Practice' *British Journal of Midwifery* 1997; **5(2):** 100–104

Sackett DL, Richardson WS, Rosenberg WMC, Haynes RB *Evidence-based Medicine: how to practice and teach EBM* London: Churchill Livingstone; 1997

Sackett DL, Rosenberg WMC, Gray JAM, Haynes RB, Richardson WS 'Evidence-based Medicine: what it is and what it isn't' *BMJ* 1996; **312:** 71–72

Sheldon TA, Guyatt GH, Haines A 'When to Act on the Evidence' *BMJ* 1998; **317:** 139–142

Smith MA 'Health Technology Assessment and the NHS R&D Initiative' *J Med Eng & Tech* 1996; **20(6):** 192–195

Straus SE, Sackett DL 'Using Research Findings in Clinical Practice' *BMJ* 1998; **317:** 339–342

4

Ethics and good practice

Hazel E McHaffie

KEY ISSUES

- Clinical and research contracts
- The basic ethical principles
- Accountability
- Responsibilities of all midwives in relation to research
- Responsibilities of midwives in managerial positions
- Additional responsibilities of researchers
- The role of Ethics Committees.

INTRODUCTION

With an increasing emphasis on public accountability, research has become an ethical imperative for midwives. Indeed, the International Code of Ethics for Midwives (International Confederation of Midwives 1993) stipulates that professionals should 'develop and share midwifery knowledge through a variety of processes such as peer review and research'.

However, research in midwifery introduces certain ethical issues which may challenge researchers as well as clinical midwives. Newborn infants are vulnerable because they cannot defend themselves. Women having babies are vulnerable too. Being protective of their babies – whether unborn or born – they are reluctant to do anything to jeopardize the care given to them. Altruism is a compelling factor when it comes to women's willingness to contribute to a research study, but they may fear the consequences for themselves or their babies. If they do not conform to a request to participate, they may fear antagonizing their carers and, in some way, receiving sub-optimal attention as a result. Furthermore, there is sometimes a perceived imbalance of power between the client and the health care professional which renders the women disadvantaged.

For all these reasons it is crucial that all those involved in research in midwifery in any capacity – the clinician implementing research every bit as much as the researcher undertaking the investigation – give careful attention to ensure that women and babies are adequately protected. This chapter focuses on the ways in which research can be designed and managed in order to maximize good and minimize harm. The ethical principles underpinning research will provide a frame of reference for a detailed consideration of good conduct.

CONTRACTS – CLINICAL AND RESEARCH

Box 4.1   Clinician and researcher: different responsibilities

Rosemary Jardin is a 23-year-old woman living with her current partner in a 13th floor flat in Wolverhampton. She has been having babies since she was 15 when her first child, a boy, was born. Four of them aged 6, 5, 3 and 2 years live with her. Jade, born at just 25 weeks, has been discharged from the Neonatal Unit. You, as the liaison midwife from the Neonatal Unit, go to visit Rosemary and Jade at home and find the baby very agitated. Over several hours you discover that the baby's skin is in poor condition and she is losing weight; hygiene leaves much to be desired; the father has left home; Rosemary is very hostile to the baby.

You are responsible clinically for following up the family on a routine basis. You will probably start to address systematically the various problems facing Rosemary and her baby and will also mobilize support. If, however, it is I, a researcher studying the follow-up management of very premature infants, who am present, there will be other priorities which complicate my response. I may want to know how adequate the existing services are, for example. If I start to interfere and change the status quo, I will have changed the experience for Rosemary and will need to remove her from my sample. This is a hard fact to assimilate: perhaps I have already visited her four times and have a rich store of data on this family. On the other hand, my native care and compassion may overrule my researcher's caution. I may come to Rosemary's aid even though I accept it will have detrimental consequences as far as my research is concerned. Perhaps, I then face the ensuing wrath of the local health visitor and GP who have been watching this family carefully, coaxing them to be self-sufficient and to tap into their own network of support. I am caught in a Catch 22 situation. How can I resolve it satisfactorily? How can I weigh the long-term benefits of the research for many other families against the short-term well-being of this one family?

The case above is illustrative of a real dilemma. It underlines the difference between the contract a researcher has with a respondent and that a midwife has with a client. It can be very difficult for a midwife, trained to identify a need and respond actively to it, to stand back and simply observe. But the quality of research depends on careful observation, thought, recording and analysis. The integrity of the research may be compromised by the need to consider the safety or well-being of the clients or respondents. When does human concern take over from researcher impartiality? When should it?

OVERALL APPROACH

Throughout all parts of the research process there are ethical decisions to be made; judgments about what is right and what is wrong. Is this an important and relevant subject to explore? Am I the right person to carry out this study? Is this the right way to go about it? Are these the right people to involve in it – staff, mothers and babies, families? Is it acceptable to report this finding? Have I protected my respondents adequately? Have the results been disseminated to all the groups who should know about them? For the most part it is relatively easy to know when a course of action becomes wrong. But where values and principles conflict then a dilemma presents, as we have seen.

All of us have our own values, beliefs and standards. Some are more highly developed than others. But wherever we are in our thinking about these matters, it is important to remember that, whether we are clinicians or researchers, whether the research is qualitative or quantitative, we are each accountable for our practice. We must be able to justify the decisions which we make. To be accountable, we must base our work on the best available evidence of good practice. Research in midwifery and in maternal–child care has been aiming to establish these gold standards. But not all research is valuable, not all research is sound. Being personally accountable involves discrimination, critically evaluating what is done in the name of science and effectively utilizing what is good (Clark 1991).

ETHICAL PRINCIPLES UNDERPINNING RESEARCH

Many people switch off at the very mention of ethics. Too often the subject is shrouded in mystery, littered with obscure, archaic terms and threatening concepts. Let's avoid all those pitfalls and go to the heart of the matter. The basic ethical principles which apply to the conduct of research in midwifery are those which also underpin clinical midwifery care. They relate to:

* doing good and not doing harm
* trust
* justice
* autonomy
* truth.

Doing good and not doing harm

Two major principles to which midwives subscribe are those of doing good to people (otherwise known as *beneficence*) and doing them no harm (*non-maleficence*). In order to uphold these principles, every individual should examine constantly their practice, monitor the effects of their actions and find better ways of providing a midwifery service which is maximally beneficial and minimally harmful. Good quality research into practice facilitates this process. For their part, researchers must also ensure that what they do does no harm. However, sometimes they cannot promise that the respondents involved in their research will receive benefit – sometimes the good lies in the application of the findings to the care of future clients. For example, I am currently carrying out a study into the experiences of families where treatment has been withdrawn from sick infants. I cannot promise the parents I recruit that the study will help them, only that the findings will be used to help other families in the future who are facing this tragedy. They have volunteered to participate anyway, because they want to help other parents so much. Participating is beneficial for them in itself; some good has come out of a very bad situation. It is an added bonus that most of them have found it therapeutic to talk in detail about their experience.

Trust

Women trust themselves to midwives in the expectation that, as professionals, they will use their skills and knowledge to good effect and care for them as well as they are able. The relationship is one of trust (based on the principle of *fidelity*). Respondents trust that researchers too will be guided by similar high principles and that the projects they are involved in will aim to improve the quality of care provided or will increase knowledge of disease and cure. Researchers, then, have an obligation to safeguard the welfare of their respondents. Preserving the participants' well-being may have consequences for the research, and may even mean abandoning data collection from certain respondents where intervention has altered the naturally occurring conditions. It may even mean abandoning the project entirely if events demonstrate that the consequences are too harmful to justify continuing. Thus, in the trial of Extra Corporeal Membrane Oxygenation (ECMO), the study came to a premature end because the benefits of the treatment to neonates were so clear that it would have been unethical to deny it to the control babies (UK Collaborative ECMO Trial Group 1996).

Justice

Women expect to be treated fairly (the principle of *justice*). In clinical practice, for instance, it would seem unfair if one mother had to provide her own sheets, towels and laundering when the woman in the adjacent bed had hers provided by the hospital. Similarly, in research there needs to be a perceived fairness. It would be unacceptable to take swabs from a woman following delivery with a cursory comment that they were needed for research purposes if you then provided a detailed explanation and leaflet about the research to another woman. Similarly, it would be unfair to ask midwives in a busy Neonatal Unit to participate in a third project after two, which had absorbed much time and energy, had recently taken place.

Autonomy

Increasingly, women are encouraged to decide for themselves and take a measure of control for what happens with and to them (respect for autonomy). Thus, for example, women in some centres complete birth plans which detail what kind of management they wish for when they go into labour and during delivery and the puerperium. In stating their preferences in this way they are helping to ensure that the experience is as they would choose, rather than putting themselves into the hands of the professionals to manage events as they think fit. In research the same principle applies. Respondents should be given the opportunity to look at the conditions of participation and choose for themselves whether these are acceptable. One mother might find it too troubling to enrol herself in a study which necessitates giving three extra blood samples during weeks 30–36 of her pregnancy. She is not obliged to enter the study and her care will be unaffected if she declines to do so. In this way, she exercises her right as an autonomous person to control her own life.

Truth

In order to make rational decisions for themselves, people need to be accurately and fully informed. Here the principle of truth-telling (*veracity*) and informed consent apply. A mother cannot make a fully autonomous choice about whether or not she wants analgesia in labour if she has no conception of the pain of labour or if she is not told about the alternative forms of pain relief available to her. Similarly, in research a mother is not in a position to give informed consent to involve her premature baby in a trial of surfactant if she has no idea of the physiology of the lungs, the effect of this specific drug or the possible consequences of either treatment or non-treatment with this substance.

ACCOUNTABILITY OF ALL MIDWIVES

Research involving women and their new babies cannot be divorced from clinical practice. If the woman and/or her baby are receiving care from midwives, then the clinical staff have duties and responsibilities towards them (UKCC 1994). The government has underlined the requirement for partnerships between researchers, clinicians and managers (Scottish Office Home and Health Department 1993). Good research depends on good co-operation and good communication.

Midwives are professionally accountable practitioners. They are instructed that: 'In all circumstances the safety and welfare of the mother and her baby must be of primary importance' (UKCC 1994). Of course, supporting research which will ultimately help in the development of a safer and more effective management of pregnancy and childbirth is part of that responsibility. But 'In all circumstances'? Even when you can see that the proposed research has a clear value for mothers or babies in the future, but it is less than beneficial to these particular mothers or babies? Even when it means you will negate 6 months of careful data collecting?

The importance of the midwife's conduct, whatever her involvement in the research process, cannot be over emphasized. For this reason the

---

Box 4.2   Research and clinical care: whose interests are paramount?

Imagine you are in charge of a postnatal ward with 30 women and their babies. A research project is proposed to examine the rate of healing of the perineum after delivery. It involves researchers measuring perineal trauma daily for 10 days.

- Would you let an unknown person examine intimately the women in your care without checking their credentials?
- Would you escort the women to the examination room without explanation or asking their permission for what was to happen?
- What responsibility would community midwives have once the women are discharged home?
- What is your responsibility in effecting co-operation across the two settings?

Imagine you are working in a Special Care Nursery. A study is ongoing looking at the rates of excretion of certain chemicals. It involves sticking bags on babies to collect urine for 3 consecutive days. It also involves not washing the baby for those 3 days, other than to cleanse with sterile water after soiling or urinating.

- Would you go along with this form of management of the babies in your care without question?
- What would you say to the mothers of these babies?
- If you have misgivings, what will you do?
- Would you challenge the senior neonatologist heading the research team?
- If not, why not?

---

discussion in this chapter about responsibilities has been divided into three different sections: all midwives, managers, and researchers. For ease of reference and for clarity, summaries are provided before more detailed explanations.

RESPONSIBILITIES OF ALL MIDWIVES IN RELATION TO RESEARCH

Summary

All midwives must:

- satisfy themselves that the research being undertaken is ethically sound and women and babies are protected
- share any misgivings with the appropriate authority
- ensure women are given full and accurate explanation of what involvement in research entails, about the potential risks and consequences of participating
- reinforce the message that women can withdraw at any time without incurring penalties
- notify the researcher and employers where research duties conflict with clinical responsibilities
- be scrupulously careful about accuracy and personal integrity
- protect confidentiality.

Detailed discussion

All midwives must:

- *satisfy themselves that the research being undertaken is ethically sound and women and babies are protected*. Research which is poorly designed or which will not produce reliable results is unethical. It should be noted that even seemingly innocuous research may have a deleterious effect. Insensitive questions can cause pain. It can lower self-esteem if a mother feels she does not know answers to questions. It may be hurtful to realize that her experience was not as good as that of other women. Long-term anxiety, dissatisfaction or distress may result. Special care should be exercised where there is commercial involvement in a trial to ensure there are no biases or unethical restrictions distorting the study.
- *share any misgivings with the appropriate authority*. If there are any doubts about the ethics of a project or the wisdom of a given person participating, midwives have a duty to voice such concerns.
- *ensure women are given full and accurate explanation of what involvement in research entails, about the potential risks and consequences of participating*. It is good practice to:
  - give information well in advance of asking women for their consent to participate. They should be able to think through the issues carefully and quietly, to ask relevant questions and perhaps consult with others.
  - ask potential recruits to consent as close to the event as possible, if the research involves being randomized to a particular group, receiving or not receiving a particular treatment.
  - provide information in writing as well as verbally so that the woman and her partner can keep it and can study it at their leisure.
  - phrase any explanations in understandable language which is informative without being patronizing
  - provide information in a form acceptable to those with particular needs, eg. women from different cultures, those who speak different languages, or who have disabilities.

It should be noted that, on occasion, the research itself will not be possible if full information is given, since such knowledge would skew the data. In such circumstances careful cost–benefit analysis and independent assessment must determine the correct action.

- *reinforce the message that women can withdraw at any time without incurring penalties*. It is also incumbent upon the midwife to ensure that the woman knows it may not be possible to withdraw from the trial past a certain point. For example, in a trial of prostaglandin gel, once the gel is inserted in the vagina it cannot be removed if the woman decides not to proceed.

- *notify the researcher and employers where research duties conflict with clinical responsibilities.* Sometimes data collection or subject recruitment present conflicts for a midwife whose prime responsibility it is to offer clinical care.
- *be scrupulously careful about accuracy and personal integrity.* If the midwife is involved in the research process in any capacity, he or she is subject to the basic ethical principles (outlined previously) which govern all those involved in research. This is in addition to responsibilities relating to clinical function.
- *protect confidentiality.* It is vital for midwives to understand that information they obtain as clinicians may not be made available to the research team and data collected for research purposes cannot be used for normal midwifery care without the express permission of the respondents and of the principal investigator (Dimond 1990).

RESPONSIBILITIES OF MIDWIVES IN MANAGERIAL POSITIONS

Summary

Managers should:

- encourage and facilitate research which will help to inform good practice
- ensure the interests of clients and staff are not compromised by the demands of the research
- respect researchers' obligation to declare that research is beyond their competence or not feasible within constraints
- be satisfied that respondents are fully informed and duly protected
- ensure service staff, employers, colleagues and sponsors respect the right to anonymity and confidentiality
- encourage and facilitate adequate reporting, dissemination and usage of research findings, irrespective of their reflection on service provision
- refrain from using discovery of aberrant practices to discipline or punish individuals.

Detailed discussion

Managers are in a position to facilitate or hinder research. They also have responsibility for the protection of those in their area of oversight and control. Therefore they need to exercise special caution in order to support research which will benefit the service but not harm others. To this end they should:

- *encourage and facilitate research which will help to inform good practice.* It is incumbent on managers to deter individuals from undertaking research which is unsound, inappropriate or beyond their resources. If managers are commissioning or sanctioning research in their area, they must ensure projects undertaken are desirable and achievable. Determining whether they are sound may necessitate seeking expert advice.

- *ensure the interests of clients and staff are not compromised by the demands of the research.* The welfare of the potential respondents comes before the needs of the research.
- *respect researchers' obligation to declare that research is beyond their competence or not feasible within constraints.* If a potential researcher admits to reservations in this way they must be heeded. They are professionally accountable and have a duty to state that the task is outwith their skills or the available resources.
- *be satisfied that respondents are fully informed and duly protected.*
- *ensure service staff, employers, colleagues and sponsors respect the right to anonymity and confidentiality.* It is difficult to ensure this requirement is respected. Managers, however, can facilitate such an ethos by setting a good example and specifically drawing attention to the issue.
- *encourage and facilitate adequate reporting, dissemination and usage of research findings, irrespective of their reflection on service provision.*
- *refrain from using discovery of aberrant practices to discipline or punish individuals.* Disclosures should be used constructively to improve practice in general and not destructively or punitively.

ADDITIONAL RESPONSIBILITIES OF RESEARCHERS

Summary

Researchers should:

- demonstrate personal integrity
  - recognize the limits of their competence and not accept or take on activities beyond their capability without guidance or expert help
  - novices should work under the supervision of experienced researchers
  - report any ways in which they, personally, may have influenced events
  - declare their identity
  - report decisions which may have altered the results in any way
  - publish findings and adequately disseminate them
  - report the truth
  - report limitations
  - acknowledge biases
  - acknowledge others' contributions
  - respect copyright regulations.

- take a responsible approach towards participants
  - ensure the information being sought is not already known
  - seek the approval of an Ethics Committee
  - gain access through appropriate protective channels
  - forewarn potential respondents of any possible risks attached to participation
  - ensure they are fully informed about what the project entails
  - ensure they know they can decline to participate or withdraw at any time without sanction
  - respect confidentiality and anonymity
  - protect the vulnerable
  - give some feedback
  - report and disseminate the results.

- take a responsible approach towards colleagues, service staff, sponsors, employers
  - recognize and make known to relevant sponsors or supervisors personal biases which may influence the research
  - make sure sponsors know that solutions to problems or advantageous results cannot be guaranteed
  - establish, document and circulate clear terms and conditions for the conduct of research so that those concerned (sponsors, employers, colleagues) are fully informed
  - ensure service staff are aware of the requirements of the research if it involves a contribution from them
  - declare to employers any conflict of interest
  - ensure all concerned are aware of and accept the terms and conditions attached to the grant which supports the research
  - alert all members of the team to particular areas of ethical importance in the conduct of the study and the need to maintain high standards at all times
  - report findings and conclusions to sponsors and colleagues
  - ensure those who are responsible for the care of respondents know they are involved in a project, even if their permission is not required.

Detailed discussion

Midwives who undertake research are clearly subject to the usual rules governing their professional behaviour. But they have additional responsibilities which, for convenience and clarity, may be divided roughly into three areas, although there are areas of overlap: matters relating to personal integrity; responsibility towards respondents; and responsibilities towards colleagues, service staff, sponsors and employers.

Personal integrity

Researchers should:

- *recognize the limits of their competence and not accept or take on activities beyond their capability without guidance or expert help.* Researchers need to make it clear to employers or sponsors if demands exceed resources – time, finances, or expertise. It is rare that one person has all the skills necessary for every part of a research process. In any case it is a matter of good practice for all researchers, no matter how experienced, to subject their work to others for scrutiny and to involve experts in the various stages of the process to ensure high standards are maintained.
- *novices should work under the supervision of experienced researchers.* Research is every bit as much a speciality as other areas of practice and it should not be thought or expected that midwives can simply pick it up as they go along.
- *report any ways in which they, personally, may have influenced events.* If the researcher has had an impact in some way on the experience of the respondents this must be declared. It may have had an effect on the validity of the findings (Hunt 1989).
- *declare their identity.* Occasionally researchers enter a research world incognito in order to gather rich data which would otherwise be largely inaccessible to them. For example, this might be done to access the worlds of criminals, homosexuals, or nursing auxiliaries. Undoubtedly the results of such studies are powerful but serious thought must be given to the rights of those being observed and those who disclose information unwittingly (Johnson 1992). Many people feel such practices are beyond the realms of what is acceptable. Careful and expert guidance should be sought if any duplicitous approaches are contemplated.
- *report decisions which may have altered the results in any way.* Sometimes burdensome and difficult choices have to be made. The Data Protection Act (1984) has set boundaries around what information may or may not be disclosed. This may limit the information which is accessible to researchers from the outset. Subsequent developments within the trial may have influenced outcomes or results; for example, a sub-group may be seriously under-represented or a question may have been ambiguous and misunderstood by respondents. All such developments should be reported in order for the reader to form an assessment of the validity of the findings.
- *publish findings and adequately disseminate them.* Many studies have never been published (Hicks 1992). When respondents have contributed time, energy and something of themselves, they are entitled to know their data have been used in the way they were told it would be. It is unethical to 'use' people in this way. Funding bodies too are entitled to tangible returns for their investment.

- *report the truth*. Researchers have to be prepared to allow access to their raw data. Any concealment breeds suspicion. Actual examples of researchers falsifying their results are relatively few but attract severe censure (e.g. Dyer 1997a, Dyer 1997b). More common is the practice of doctoring reporting to sanitize the process. Not only is this intellectually dishonest, but it also carries a risk that others will repeat the errors. It is crucial that results which do not support an hypothesis or hunch should be reported as well as those which do. The exceptions to the majority view must be noted and the alternative explanations of a finding offered to balance the researcher's own preferred interpretation.
- *report limitations*. No research project conducted in the natural world is perfect. To pretend that it was is to risk losing credibility and to compromise one's personal integrity. Far better to acknowledge the slow recruitment which limited the final sample size, the unexpected hitches in gaining access to respondents, the choice of inappropriate tools or the constraints of real life situations.
- *acknowledge biases*. Biases may come from within the research team or from without. A personal interest in a topic may lead some researchers to select a particular area to research; for example, Glaser & Strauss (1966) chose to study the dying process after watching close relatives die. This is not necessarily a bad thing but it should be declared so that the reader can assess whether or not it had an untoward bias. Outside biases may come from the host organization or the funding body. Thus a hospital's administrators might judge that disclosure of a particular part of the findings might seriously harm the morale of its staff: they might determine that the benefit to the researcher of full reporting is of less value than the greater good of service staff. Funding bodies may resist the publication of some results if they reflect adversely on a drug or a service. In such cases careful negotiation will be required and impartial expert advice should be sought to ensure that the most ethical decision is made.
- *acknowledge others' contributions*. It is a matter of courtesy to pay tribute to the contribution made by others, e.g. funding for a project; laborious transcription of taped interviews or collection of specimens. Unfortunately preserving anonymity or confidentiality sometimes imposes restrictions on what may be specified and acknowledgements may have to be general rather than specific. Due recognition extends to the written and spoken word and where others' work is being quoted the source must be acknowledged. Plagiarism is always unacceptable.
- *respect copyright regulations*.

Responsibility to participants

Researchers should:

- ensure the information being sought is not already known.

- *seek the approval of an Ethics Committee.* This is essential if women or babies are involved, in order to ensure they are adequately protected. If the respondents are professional staff, advice should be sought from the local Health Authority/Board as requirements vary (see chapter 14).
- *gain access through appropriate protective channels.* It is easy for a researcher to feel the importance of their study warrants wholehearted support. Sometimes, however, potential respondents need protection. They may have been overly involved in research in the recent past or there may be demands on them from other sources. It is both necessary and desirable that managers with an overview of events in their area should have knowledge of proposed studies in order to offer such protection.
- *forewarn potential respondents of any possible risks attached to participation.* Hazards of radioactive substances or aggressive drug regimes are obvious. Less well recognized are the emotional, psychological and social harms which may attend participation in some studies. Being assigned to a control group where one does not get an attractive-sounding treatment or being questioned about socially unacceptable practices can leave a respondent feeling undermined and dissatisfied.
- *ensure they are fully informed about what the project entails.* Permission should be recorded formally unless the project simply involves return of a questionnaire, in which case response indicates consent. Where there are particularly sensitive issues at stake, it can be wise to seek the advice of a legal expert in drafting an appropriate document. Some Ethics Committees require use of their standard forms. On occasion it may be impossible to be totally frank with respondents if accurate information is to be obtained. For example, if you wish to know how women respond to the support provided by different individuals in a health care team, knowing exactly what factors are under investigation could well influence the behaviour of both mother and professionals. The explanation then should be couched in terms which are sufficiently clear as to be accurate, without betraying the specific focus of the study. In order to obtain certain kinds of information it might be necessary to observe behaviours without the respondents knowing that they are being watched (e.g. to detect the incidence of child abuse in hospital). Such covert practices infringe people's right to privacy and expert guidance and ongoing supervision should be sought if they are contemplated (Hicks 1996).
- *ensure they know they can decline to participate or withdraw at any time without sanction.* This right must be respected and no attempt made to coerce respondents into changing their minds. It is all too easy for vulnerable clients to feel beholden and afraid to decline.
- *respect confidentiality and anonymity.* A particular point which seems to need reinforcement is that permission is required to use information held in notes and records. Data should be treated as confidential and

only shared with members of the research team on the basis of a need to know. Sometimes it may become necessary to disclose important information which indicates a risk to the respondent or to others. Dilemmas can present and it can be very burdensome to be in receipt of such information (McHaffie 1996). The risks and benefits of breaking confidences must be weighed up carefully. Whenever possible, the respondent should be notified of any intention to reveal the disclosure. A wise precaution is to establish lines of communication before such a situation arises and build in not only an agreed procedure but support for the researcher in such an event.

- *protect the vulnerable.* Researchers must be alert to the potential to exploit relationships with an inherent inequality. The most vulnerable – the student keen to please a teacher or the disadvantaged mother anxious to conform to accepted behaviour – may agree to participate against their better judgement because of unseen pressures.
- *give some feedback.* Research respondents give of themselves through their participation in projects. They deserve some sort of feedback once the findings are analysed. In some cases it may even be beneficial to seek critical comment from them about preliminary results to strengthen the conclusions and recommendations which emerge.
- *report and disseminate the results.* It is unacceptable to conduct a study and fail to report what was found. Disseminating the findings and recommendations for practice is a part of the research process which researchers should build into their protocols from the outset.

Responsibility to colleagues, service staff, sponsors, employers

Researchers should:

- *recognize and make known to relevant sponsors or supervisors personal biases which may influence the research.*
- *make sure sponsors know that solutions to problems or advantageous results cannot be guaranteed.*
- *establish, document and circulate clear terms and conditions for the conduct of research so that those concerned (sponsors, employers, colleagues) are fully informed.* Setting out definite terms for operating can help to avoid later misunderstandings. I lived to regret not specifying what a 'full report' would entail when some of my respondents expressed unease following publication of the report by a professional publishing house.
- *ensure service staff are aware of the requirements of the research if it involves a contribution from them.*
- *declare to employers any conflict of interest.* There may, on occasion, be a tension between commitment to the research and the demands of clinical practice which employers should be fully aware of.
- *ensure all concerned are aware of and accept the terms and conditions attached*

to the grant which supports the research. Researchers have responsibilities to funding agencies to meet the terms of their agreements. If it becomes necessary for any reason to deviate from the study protocol, for example if recruitment is slower than expected; if a procedure cannot be followed because of limitations in the clinical setting, such changes should be notified to the funders. This will allow them to assess the value of the revised study and to suggest any course of action they require. Sometimes grant-giving bodies impose their own embargoes, for example on certain findings or on the extent of publishing. In such cases all concerned should be aware of these restrictions and form their own assessment of the ethical acceptability of being involved.

- *alert all members of the team to particular areas of ethical importance in the conduct of the study and the need to maintain high standards at all times.*
- *report findings and conclusions to sponsors and colleagues.*
- *ensure those who are responsible for the care of respondents know they are involved in a project, even if their permission is not required.* I have made it a practice to inform GPs (and sometimes Health Visitors too) when their patients are participating in my studies. This seems to be a matter of common courtesy when they are responsible for the overall health of these individuals.

Box 4.3 Guidelines

Recommendations for an ethical approach to research have been drawn up by a number of different organizations (e.g. World Medical Association latest revision 1989, Ethics Advisory Committee British Paediatric Association 1992, Standing Joint Committee of the British Paediatric Association and the Royal College of Obstetricians and Gynaecologists 1993, Royal College of Nursing 1998, Royal College of Physicians 1996, Association for Improvements in the Maternity Services and The National Childbirth Trust Undated). These are very variable in quality and comprehensiveness, but their range and detail demonstrate how seriously these matters are viewed. Midwives can draw on all such documents but a more specific focus is useful.

THE ROLE OF ETHICS COMMITTEES

Box 4.4 Researcher or Ethics Committee: Who should decide on limits?

You read a report of a study in which a clinical midwife undertaking research scrutinized the notes of 3500 women who had delivered within the preceding year in her place of work – the local maternity hospital. The investigation involved selecting families who a) came from areas of multiple disadvantage and b) failed to attend parentcraft classes. These parents were then interviewed (using tape recordings) in their own homes by the researcher who asked questions about childrearing and feeding; resumption of sexual activity; and access to GPs, Health Visitors and Social Workers. There is no mention of the protocol having been submitted to an Ethics Committee. What questions would this raise in your mind?

Local Research Ethics Committees exist for the scrutiny of proposed research projects to ensure both clients and researchers are adequately protected. Each Health Authority (Health Board in Scotland) is required to set up appropriately constituted committees (Royal College of Physicians 1996, Department of Health 1991, Scottish Office Home and Health Department 1992). Some institutions add additional internal systems of scrutiny. Committees vary in their structure and way of operating and intending researchers should obtain information about the requirements of the relevant Committee from their local Health Authority/Board.

These Committees have a duty to ensure that any decisions made are ethical; respondents are fully informed as far as possible and where this is not possible their interests are adequately safeguarded; that they have the capacity to give informed consent; that the wording of any documentation is understandable and sensitive; that the study does not present unreasonable demands or risks; that individual are protected against esoteric programmes designed to boost egos, further political ends or advance professional careers. Their independent scrutiny should be seen as a helpful safeguard rather than an unnecessary hurdle to be overcome. Guidance on applying for ethics approval is given in Chapter 14.

CONCLUSION

Carrying out research is a privilege not a right. Respondents may render themselves vulnerable by participating; clinical colleagues may have their work impeded, their security ruffled; institutions may run the risk of exposure to criticism or unrest. And yet both clients and staff may benefit greatly from well conducted research. Clinicians need sound answers to the questions which underlie practice; with such knowledge they can offer the best care possible to mothers and babies.

Scrupulous personal integrity, coupled with a healthy respect for others, is the hallmark of good research. If all concerned are careful to protect the mothers and babies, and colleagues, as well as to ensure only good, usable, feasible projects are undertaken, then there is less scope for inappropriate projects to get off the starting blocks or unethical breaches of conduct to be introduced. Once a suitable project is selected, researchers and clinical midwives, by asking the difficult questions at each stage of the research process, can establish the most ethical way to proceed. They each bring different values and experiences to the consideration. By respecting the other's contribution and working side by side, challenging healthily, scrutinizing effectively, clinicians and researchers can together help to provide a sounder basis for practice.

Box 4.5   Personal reflection or discussion

1. Imagine you are researching the practices of three groups of midwives who provide bereavement care for families whose babies died in a Neonatal Unit. In one of the teams you find a midwife who is reported by several respondents to be less than supportive to families from socially deprived backgrounds. In the safety of a confidential interview her professional colleagues confirm that she has strongly negative views about such families. What will you do about such information?

2. You are carrying out a randomized controlled trial of a new version of prophylactic Vitamin K for neonates. After randomization, 23 of the 105 women in the experimental arm of your study say they are no longer willing to have the treatment given to their babies because they have just watched a TV programme which suggested that any medication given to babies in the first 3 days of life is potentially harmful. Ten others whose infants received the vitamin during the previous 4 days 'phone you, very distressed because they feel they and you have put their child at risk. How will you manage this development?

3. You are keen to study the impact of a male midwife in an area of great ethnic and cultural diversity. What points would you take into account in designing such a study?

4. You are investigating the responses of fathers to their new infants. In confidence, a mother tells you that her baby is actually the product of artificial insemination by donor and the man she lives with is not the biological father. You have only 20 fathers in your study so this one family represents 5% of your total sample. How will you deal with reporting of this information?

5. You have a close friend with AIDS who has recently had a baby. Since she found she was pregnant she has been telling you about her experiences of being isolated and stigmatized. Incensed by her less than optimal care, you determine to design a study to find out how HIV positive pregnant women are treated. What factors might you build into the enquiry to minimize subjectivity and bias?

FURTHER READING

Reports of ethically questionable research
Josefson D 'US Journal Attacks Unethical HIV Trials' *British Medical Journal* 1997; **314:** 765
Mudur G 'Indian study of Women with Cervical Lesions Called Unethical' *British Medical Journal* 1997; **314:** 1065
Wise J, 'Karolinska Professor Broke Research Rules' *British Medical Journal* 1997; **314:** 536
Wise J 'Research Suppressed for Seven Years by Drug Company' *British Medical Journal* 1997; **314:** 1145
Wise J 'AIDS drug trials attacked' *British Medical Journal* 1997; **314:** 1224

Issues underlying research in sensitive areas
Renzetti CM, Lee RL *Researching Sensitive Topics* California: Sage; 1993
McIlaffie HE 'Researching Sensitive Issues' In Frith L, Ed. *Ethics and Midwifery. Issues in Contemporary Practice* Oxford: Butterworth-Heinemann; 1996 pp.258–273

Ethical problems
Hicks C, 'Ethics in Midwifery Research' In Frith L, Ed. *Ethics and Midwifery. Issues in Contemporary Practice* Oxford: Butterworth-Heinemann; 1996

Trickery and withholding of information
Bakhurst D, 'On Lying and Deceiving' *Journal of Medical Ethics* 1992; **18:** 63–66
Jackson J, 'On the Morality of Deception – does method matter? A reply to David Bakhurst' *Journal of Medical Ethics* 1993; **19:** 183–187

REFERENCES

Association for Improvements in the Maternity Services and The National Childbirth Trust *A Charter for Ethical Research in Maternity Care* London: AIMS & NCT: undated

Clark E *Evaluating Research* Module 10 in Research Awareness programme London: Distance Learning Centre South Bank Polytechnic; 1991

Department of Health *Local Research Ethics Committees* London: HMSO; 1991

Dimond B 'Legal Aspects of Research' *Nursing Standard* 1990; **4(39):** 44–46

Dyer C 'Consultant Struck off Over Research Fraud' *British Medical Journal* 1997a; **314:** 205

Dyer C 'ME Researcher Accused of Cooking the Books' *British Medical Journal* 1997b; **314:** 271

Ethics Advisory Committee, British Paediatric Association. *Guidelines for the Ethical Conduct of Medical Research Involving Children* London: BPA; 1992

Glaser BG, Strauss AL *Awareness of Dying* Chicago: Aldine Publishing Company; 1966

Hicks C 'Research in Midwifery: Are midwives their own worst enemies?' *Midwifery* 1992; **8:** 12–18

Hicks C 'Ethics in Midwifery Research' In *Ethics and Midwifery. Issues in Contemporary Practice* Frith L Oxford: Butterworth Heinemann; 1996, pp 237–257

Hunt JC *Psychoanalytical Aspects of Fieldwork* London: Sage; 1989

International Confederation of Midwives *International Code of Ethics for Midwives* Geneva: ICM; 1993

Johnson M A silent conspiracy? Some ethical issues of participant observation in nursing research. *International Journal of Nursing Studies*, 1992; 29; **2:** 213–223

McHaffie HE 'Researching sensitive issues' In Frith L *Ethics and Midwifery. Issues in Contemporary Practice* Oxford: Butterworth-Heinemann; 1996, pp 258–273

Royal College of Nursing *Ethics related to Research in Nursing* Middlesex; Scutari: 1998

Royal College of Physicians *Guidelines on the Practice of Ethics Committees in Medical Research Involving Human Subjects* Third edition London: RCP; 1996

Scottish Office Home and Health Department *Local Research Ethics Committees* Scotland: HMSO; 1992

Scottish Office Home and Health Department *Research and Development Strategy for the National Health Service in Scotland* Edinburgh: CSO; 1993

Standing Joint Committee of the British Paediatric Association and the Royal College of Obstetricians and Gynaecologists *A Checklist of Questions to Ask When Evaluating Proposed Research During Pregnancy and Following Birth* London: BPA & RCOG; 1993

UK Collaborative ECMO Trial Group 'UK collaborative randomized trial of neonatal extracorporeal membrane oxygenation' *Lancet* 1996; **348:** 75–82

United Kingdom Central Council for Nursing, Midwifery and Health Visiting *The Midwife's Code of Practice* London: UKCC; 1994

World Medical Association *Declaration of Helsinki* Royal Medical Association; 1975

5

Involving consumers in research

Elisabeth Buggins and Mary Nolan

KEY ISSUES

- How can health services consumers in general, and women and their families in particular, participate in research into maternity care to ensure that their needs are its focus?
- What stages of the research

  process can they be involved in?
- What are the barriers to involving them?
- How can these barriers be broken down?
- How can consumers help to disseminate research findings?

INTRODUCTION

'The involvement of consumers in research changes the priorities for research. Simply having consumers present at research meetings can have a powerful effect – they remind researchers of the purpose of their work.' (First Report of the Standing Advisory Group on Consumer Involvement in the NHS Research and Development Programme 1996/7)

The Standing Advisory Group on Consumer Involvement was convened by the Central Research and Development Committee of the NHS Research and Development Programme in April 1996. The quotation above is taken from the Introduction to its First Report. The Central Research Committee is advised by four Standing Groups and the fact that one of these should be devoted entirely to ensuring that consumers influence every stage of the research programme reflects ongoing changes in government and popular thinking. It also demonstrates the gradual movement away from a positivistic model of health care, which reduces each individual to a sequence of bio-chemical reactions, and towards an holistic model, which acknowledges that the client's own perception of her needs should be crucial in determining the kind of care she receives and the manner in which it is delivered.

Maternity care has been in the vanguard of new developments influencing the experience of care generally in the late twentieth century. Four years before the Standing Advisory Group on Consumer Involvement began its work, Nicholas Winterton's seminal Report on the Maternity Services (House of Commons 1992) dedicated itself to exploring and making transparent 'what desires women express in terms of a responsive and appropriate maternity service (compared with) what they actually experience.'

Its focus on the relevance and centrality of the insights of women who have used the maternity services was enshrined in the First Principle of Good Maternity Care in the Report of the Expert Maternity Group which followed Winterton's Report:

'The woman must be the focus of maternity care. She should be able to feel that she is in control of what is happening to her ...' (Expert Maternity Group 1993)

This chapter recognizes as axiomatic the power of women and their families to change the maternity services in accordance with the vision of *A Guide to Effective Care in Pregnancy and Childbirth* (Enkin et al 1995):

'Once a critical mass of mothers becomes aware of the fact that options are available to them, major changes in obstetrical practice may ensue.' (authors' underlining)

WHY INVOLVE WOMEN IN RESEARCH INTO THE MATERNITY SERVICES?

It is very probable that midwives reading this book will not feel that this question requires an answer. Midwives work 'with women' – that is what 'midwife' means. So, midwives are well used to involving women in their work. However, for many years the traditional research agenda has been guided by a focus on specific physiological or pathological processes which have been seen as separate from the complex individual who houses these processes. Cartesian dualism, which views the body operating independently of the mind, has historically informed western thinking about medicine and care for the last 400 years. It is a view which has been challenged only recently. Attempts to encourage health professionals to work in multidisciplinary teams and to recognize the range of clients' needs, from the physical to the social, cultural, psychological and spiritual, acknowledge that health care is more complex than is allowed for within the Cartesian or scientific tradition.

It is useful for midwives to be able to put into words their innate, professional understanding of the importance of involving women in research, so that they can convince funding bodies, ethical committees and colleagues of its importance as well.

Iain Chalmers, a significant instigator of the move towards evidence-based practice, stresses that lay people draw on different kinds of knowledge and perspectives from those of professional researchers (Chalmers 1995). One of Oliver & Buchanan's informants (1997) comments that consumers are often 'a catalyst for new ways of looking at something that those of us who are more formally involved in research and implementation often forget'.

What professionals feel is of concern to women may be considerably off target when compared to what women feel is of concern to them. In this respect, Smith & Armstrong's study (1989) of consumers' requirements of General Practitioner services is interesting. The findings were that the criteria for good practice identified by the medical profession were not highly valued by patients. Where doctors rated health promotion activities highly and the ability to change easily to a different GP, patients were much more interested in having a doctor who listened to them, in having the same doctor at each appointment and in doctors who sorted out their problems. Comparing the perceptions of childbearing women and midwives, Proctor (1998) found key differences between the two in relation to a variety of aspects of the maternity service and concluded:

'Understanding exactly where the gaps exist between maternity staff and childbearing women is ... important for developing internal marketing and for gaining information on which to base risk management strategies.'

Chalmers (1995) found that consumers are more open-minded than professionals about which research questions are worth addressing, which treatment outcomes matter and what aspects of care are important; their involvement results in research that is more relevant and reliable, and more likely to be used (NHS Executive 1997).

Entwistle et al (1998) remind us of the democratic right of those who pay for the health services and for research into it – namely health service consumers – to have a say in what kinds of research are funded. Involving consumers in research may enable researchers to reach parts of the community which are normally hard to reach (Oliver & Buchanan 1997). Consumer networks may extend to individuals and whole groups of people whom health care professionals would rarely see.

Finally, it is the unique knowledge of local circumstances, of lay values and priorities and the enthusiasm and committedness of consumers in pursuing answers to the questions that are important to them which make them ideal participants in research programmes.

INPUT AT WHAT STAGE IN THE RESEARCH?

At every stage is the simple answer to this question. Consumers can be involved in determining which are the really important issues in treatment and care from their point of view and what, therefore, should be the subject of research. Consumers are also ideally placed to advise on the outcome measures for research; their perception of a beneficial outcome may be very different from that of an obstetrician, anaesthetist or even midwife (Kelson 1995).

Hope (1995) considers that consumers should be involved in choosing the focus for systematic reviews of research studies and in informing conclusions from those reviews. This is vital because 'the conclusions reached will depend on the values of the reviewers. The patient's perspective is therefore needed in drawing a final conclusion from the review'.

Involvement at the planning stage

Consumers may enable research to be more effective by offering advice at the planning stage, when thought is being given to methods for recruitment of members of the target group. Consumers may understand better than professionals what motivates people to take part. Oliver & Buchanan (1997) describe how parents were invited to help plan the ECMO (Extracorporeal Membrane Oxygenation) trial, a research study which, because it involved looking at the needs of very sick babies, demanded special sensitivity on the part of the researchers.

'Voluntary groups were invited to share with researchers and health professionals the task of deciding how the trial might best be explained to parents and how parents should be invited to allow their baby to enter the trials and how they should be supported.'

Involvement in data collection

Consumers can also be involved at the data collection stage of research. Renfrew & McCandlish (1992) describe how breastfeeding counsellors from the National Childbirth Trust were successfully involved in recruiting women into the MAIN trial (Multi-centre, Randomized Controlled Trial of Alternative Treatments for Inverted and Non-protractile Nipples in Pregnancy). NPEU (National Perinatal Epidemiology Unit) researchers approached the headquarters of the NCT to ask for assistance in the trial. The NCT's national magazine and the local branch newsletters were used to advertise the trial. Eighteen volunteer local co-ordinators were recruited from NCT's breastfeeding counsellors to check the eligibility criteria of the women who offered to participate, randomize them into a trial group and give them instructions about their allocation. As a result of the NCT's involvement, more women were recruited into a trial where recruitment was difficult, thus increasing the sample size and adding to the strength of the conclusions that could be drawn from analysis of the data.

Involvement in audit

User involvement in medical audit is increasingly seen, not merely as desirable, but as essential. Not only does the perspective of users enable service providers and health professionals to remain focused on the issues which will really make a difference to patients' and clients' experience of care, but user involvement may also protect health professionals:

'Users are less likely to demand ineffective (though "fashionable") treatments or

procedures if they are informed through involvement in the auditing process.'
(Joule 1992)

The ASQUAM (Achieving Sustainable Quality in Maternity) project based at North Staffordshire Maternity Unit works towards devising audit guidelines for different aspects of care and treatment in pregnancy and childbirth. Clinicians and service users are brought together for an annual conference to decide the areas in which it is most important to produce such guidelines. Consumers invited to attend speak favourably of an atmosphere at the conference which makes them feel that their views are heard and are considered as valid as those of the professional representatives (NHS Executive 1997).

Involvement in dissemination of findings

Involving consumers in the dissemination of research is also vital if health education objectives are to be achieved. It is only by raising levels of consciousness within the community that women can benefit from research aimed at improving the quality of the maternity services. Through knowledge, they find empowerment to challenge their own care at the individual level and public policy at the national level. Voluntary organizations and local groups have networks which are effective in spreading the results of research studies, such as the *New Generation* publication from the NCT. It is not sufficient just to publish research in professional journals where it will be accessed only by professional colleagues; equally important is to publish the results in the newsletters of local groups and in the magazines of larger charities and voluntary organizations. These publications speak directly to and for the consumer.

HOW TO ACCESS CONSUMERS AND THEIR VIEWS

Consider how you would feel if you were asked, as a community midwife, to sit on a research group composed of 20 obstetricians, health services managers and lecturers in midwifery education. Unless you are particularly confident and assertive, you would probably be far too intimidated to speak up or perhaps even to attend the meetings. The kind of tokenism whereby a single consumer is invited to attend research meetings with high-powered health professionals and researchers is very unlikely to achieve the outcome of identifying consumers' needs. One consumer is unlikely to be representative of an entire client group, such as women using the maternity services.

It has been found that standard letters are not particularly effective for seeking information about consumers' priorities (Oliver & Buchanan 1997). Just as health professionals are only beginning to get used to the idea of involving consumers in research, so consumers need a great deal of support in the brave new world of working with us. Letters not followed up by contact with a key person to explain the reason for the approach, to define what is being requested of the consumer or consumer group, to clarify the time-scale for a response and to make the offer of ongoing support and clarification as needed, are not likely to elicit a speedy response or any response at all.

Consulting with groups of consumers

In order to hear the voice of consumers, it is more effective to consult them in groups. Focus groups, in which a small number of say 6 to 12 people with relevant experience and knowledge are brought together with a skilled facilitator to exchange views about the service and to generate ideas for research or about a particular research topic, can open up a rich seam of ideas. The group's discussion can be taped (with the permission of the participants) for analysis afterwards. Fleming & Golding (1997) outline the use of focus groups:

• To find out how users experience services.
• To understand users' views, attitudes and expectations.
• As preliminary work in the preparation of a survey.
• To gauge reactions to proposed changes.

The National Childbirth Trust collaborated with North Essex Health Authority and the Mid-Essex Community Health Council to investigate what options, information and care women giving birth in the area required. Four public meetings were held in North Essex to gain information about the local maternity services. These meetings included users working on Maternity Service Liaison Committees (MSLCs), community and hospital-based midwives, a bereavement counsellor, NCT antenatal teachers and breastfeeding counsellors, representatives of consumer organizations and members of the public. In addition, focus group discussions were arranged with particular groups to seek to understand the experiences of black mothers, bereaved mothers, mothers who had had a baby in the Special Care Unit, mothers whose husbands were in the army, very young mothers, mothers on income support, disabled mothers and mothers from the traveller community (Gready et al 1995).

Consulting with MSLCs and Community Health Councils (CHCs)

User members of MSLCs and CHCs may be able to speak for groups of people using the health care services, although Kelson (1995) has questioned the representativeness of CHC members. Nonetheless, CHCs have a track record in co-ordinating the views of consumers in relation to women's health issues and have considerable experience of working both with interest groups and with providers of services.

Consulting with individual consumers

Individual interviews with women who are potential users of the maternity service, who are currently using it or who have recently used it, can be carried out to determine what aspects of the service are of most concern to them. Sometimes, women who have had particularly significant experiences (identified perhaps because they have initiated a complaints procedure) can be invited to discuss these, in order to identify those facets of care which merit immediate managerial attention and/or research investigation (*critical incident technique*). Interviewing is a skilful procedure and midwives will find it helpful to consult up-to-date texts such as Mays & Pope (1996) and talk to academics involved in research to gain an understanding of what is required.

National organizations often have funds which can be allocated for research, and midwives seeking monies for a study could consider inviting one of these to work with them, to provide ideas for research or to comment on an existing proposal. These organizations may also offer to approach contacts to assist in data collection and may suggest methods of disseminating results. Professional groups could join forces with lay groups to bid for research monies after identifying a research agenda that truly reflects the interests of both parties.

CHALLENGES TO INVOLVING CONSUMERS IN RESEARCH

Health professionals may fear that consumers will not prioritize research topics in the same way that they themselves would and that consumers will wish to pursue topics which are difficult to investigate using the quantitative methodologies favoured by the most prestigious journals.

'The involvement of consumers may change the priorities for research. There is concern amongst some professionals that involving consumers in research may divert attention away from what they – the professionals – see as the most urgent problems to be addressed.' (NHS Executive 1998)

Midwives, however, are unlikely to find themselves at variance with the research agenda set by women and their families, as the agenda is often concerned with issues around satisfaction with the birth, self-care, social support, and the experience of early parenting. These are areas with which midwives, whose focus is on the healthy woman, will probably be in considerable sympathy. It is vital that both consumers and health professionals know *why* consumers have been invited to participate in the research process; involvement merely for political correctness will satisfy nobody.

'An agreed understanding of the rationale for involving lay people and their role in a project is a prerequisite for attracting appropriate lay people, securing their commitment and making best use of their skills.' (Oliver 1996)

In order to involve consumers effectively in research, it is essential that the agenda for the research is clear from the start, that everyone knows what outcome measures are being investigated, that the roles of consumers and health professionals are clarified and that methods to incorporate the results of the research into practice are identified. If it is likely that getting the results into practice will be a lengthy process, consumers need to understand this. McIver (1995) discusses ethical issues around the briefing of consumers: 'Research ... may raise expectations that are not easily fulfilled. A frequent misunderstanding is that doing research automatically leads to implementation' (Department of Health 1995).

McIver stresses the importance of helping consumers to understand the time scale involved in research, in order to avoid disillusionment and possible future refusal to co-operate. Oliver & Buchanan (1997) advocate 'a businesslike approach with voluntary organizations enabled to contribute rather than swamped with tasks they cannot manage'.

There is no quick way to involve consumers, especially if their voice is being accessed through local or national organizations. The National Childbirth Trust has a research network of NCT members working in its 380 local Branches (Gyte 1994). However, these members are nearly always the mothers of very young children and consulting their views, or asking them to participate in gathering data, is inevitably time consuming. Renfrew and McCandlish (1992) comment on the impact of Christmas and school holidays on recruitment via NCT volunteers into the MAIN trial. One of the lessons learned from South and West Devon's experience of setting up Parent Panels was 'do not arrange parent panel meetings in July, August or December' (Matthews 1998). Health professional researchers need to take time to understand how the organization with which they are working communicates with its members and the kind of commitment they can expect from volunteers. Similarly, consumers need to be helped to understand how professional researchers organize research and what their time scale is. The key to this is good communication: consumers involved in research need to have easy access to researchers through an identified key person who understands their organization and concerns, and who has the time to answer queries. It is very unhelpful if the key person keeps changing, especially since it is the nature of voluntary organizations that their key persons change regularly. Frequent changes of personnel on both sides leads to research chaos!

It goes without saying that, for success in collaborative research between consumers and health professionals, there must be mutual respect for each other's knowledge, skills and commitment. Consumers may fear that the use of medical and research terminology will prevent them from participating fully at meetings and that their own non-technical discourse will appear ignorant and amateurish. These anxieties can be assuaged if consumers are fully briefed before meetings with papers backed up by explanations written in accessible language. Explaining to someone outside the health professions what is meant by a particular piece of jargon or how to interpret the results of a complex research paper is an excellent way of ensuring that you know what you are talking about!

Enabling consumers

When consumers are unwilling to participate in research, it is important to ask what practical issues may be preventing them from coming forward. The timing of meetings may need to be adjusted to ensure that the targeted consumers can attend. There may be financial problems to address – not everyone can afford the transport costs involved in attending a patient participation group at the local hospital. Women with young families may need assistance with child care costs or, alternatively, to be offered a creche where their children can be cared for. It may be important to make databases available to consumers to help them understand what research has already been carried out in the field under scrutiny.

Consumers may need educational, as well as practical, support if they are to maximize their contribution to a research project. Particular initiatives that have been taken to increase the ability of consumers to inform the health care debate are the CASP (critical appraisal skills programme) and VOICES projects. Researchers are increasingly aware that 'effective (and credible) use of evidence requires explicit, reproducible and efficient assessment of the evidence by a wide range of people, not all of whom may be trained in the use of biomedical literature' (Milne 1995).

Training consumers and professionals together

CASP workshops help health service decision-makers, a group which should include consumers, develop skills in appraising evidence about clinical effectiveness. Learning outcomes include:

- a better understanding of different ways of testing whether health treatments work
- being able to explain why critical appraisal is important
- knowing who to contact to discuss critical appraisal
- having the knowledge to help raise awareness of sources of information about treatment outcomes (CASP Workshop Pack 1996).

The core funding for the programme came from Anglia and Oxford

Regional Health Authority and workshops are typically attended by public health and epidemiology researchers, public health medicine doctors, non-medical managers, audit staff, health promotion officers, clinical staff and lay people. Combining people from different backgrounds is seen by the organizers as one of the advantages of the workshops (Milne 1995). Such workshops empower consumers to enter the research arena on a basis of equality with health professionals.

The VOICES project was devised and developed by the National Childbirth Trust in order to increase the confidence of lay members of Maternity Service Liaison Committees. Workshops introduce participants to the structure of the health service in general and of the maternity service in particular. They help participants to understand where and how decisions are made about local maternity care issues, and also strengthen assertiveness, communication and negotiation skills. This ensures that the voice of users is clearly heard. In particular, the project has tried to offer training to very young mothers and to mothers from ethnic minority backgrounds, to encourage them to take up positions on MSLCs so that the concerns of their groups can be addressed. Lay members of MSLCs are well placed to identify key consumer issues in maternity care. In addition, the fact that they are already accustomed to meeting with health professionals may mean that there are fewer barriers to overcome if they are invited to participate in research.

Kelson (1995) points out that it is not only consumers who need education and training in the skills necessary for research; there is also a place for educating health professionals in the attitudes which will enable consumer involvement.

'Training should cover a variety of topics including awareness training, use of language, valuing others' opinions, taking time to explain and giving space to people, and looking at their own fears and prejudices.'

GETTING RESEARCH INTO THE COMMUNITY

If consumer groups have been invited to participate in research, it is, of course, essential that the results of the research are fed back to them. This may take the form of conferences to which consumers and health professionals are invited, co-authored articles in professional and lay journals and presentations to those immediately involved in the research.

Consumers have a vital role to play in transmitting the results of research to the community. Researchers need to consider the networks available to them to disseminate their studies through newsletters, journals and magazines produced by local and national self-help groups and voluntary organizations. The National Childbirth Trust's members' magazine, New Generation, includes with each issue a Digest which aims to keep key workers, such as trained antenatal teachers, breastfeeding counsellors and postnatal exercise and discussion leaders, abreast of research and debate in their areas of work. *Changing Childbirth Update*, the newsletter published by the Changing Childbirth Implementation Team, set up in the wake of the Expert Maternity Group's Report in 1993, was distributed to key members of maternity organizations and lay representatives on MSLCs, as well as midwives, obstetricians and health service managers. It included news about research being undertaken by health professionals in maternity care, research which involved collaboration between professionals and consumers and research undertaken by voluntary organizations. This approach made it clear that valuable research is carried on in many different arenas and is not only the province of the professional researcher.

Informed Choice

Significant advances towards making research available to women on their own terms have been made by the Midwives' Information and Research Service's *Informed Choice* leaflets. These were piloted by asking women to complete questionnaires regarding the design and content of two leaflets and by carrying out some in-depth interviews with women before and after they had given birth. The questions addressed by the pilot study were:

- Was sufficient information available in the leaflets?
- Were the leaflets accessible to all women?
- Was the information read and understood by all women?

Results from the survey and interviews were used to revise the leaflets already produced and to improve the accessibility of future leaflets. Some key points emerged in terms of how best to communicate research to consumers. Pictures and diagrams are important to reinforce and elucidate the text. The written word should be backed up with face-to-face dis-

---

Box 5.1   How to go about involving consumers in your research

1. Use existing consumer networks.
2. Make personal contact by 'phone or visit; letters are often ineffective.
3. Allow sufficient time for setting up meetings and for recruitment of subjects.
4. Provide accessible briefings for consumers involved in your research and agree clear and inclusive objectives with them.
5. Ask consumers what they need in order to be able to participate comfortably and effectively in your research.
6. Budget to support travel and child care costs of consumers involved in your research.
7. Avoid data collection periods coinciding with religious festivals and school holidays. Any meetings may need to be within school hours.
8. Keep consumers informed of progress and outcomes.
9. Evaluate the process of involving consumers in your research so as to be able to inform future collaborative initiatives.

cussion – consumers like the chance to discuss leaflets with a health professional. Therefore, health professionals who are disseminating leaflets must familiarize themselves with their content and purpose before they give them out to consumers (NHS Centre for Reviews and Dissemination Report 7 1996).

FUTURE DIRECTIONS

One of the principal beneficial outcomes of consumer involvement in research is the quality of the partnership that is fostered between consumers, consumer groups, health professionals and researchers. Successful collaboration will start to break down some of the barriers which have disempowered consumers and prevented them from asking the questions that are relevant to them. Health professionals are listening to consumers to find out what aspects of care and treatment are really important to their clients:

'Today, people ... expect to feel more in control of their situation than was the case in the past. They get that not only by being given information about their condition, the treatments and services available, but also by being listened to.' (LMCA: A New Partnership, undated)

Evaluate the collaboration

It is important to recognize that the end point of research which involves consumers has not been reached when the results are disseminated, or even when they are fully incorporated into practice. There is a need to evaluate the process by which consumers were involved in the research

---

Box 5.2 Learning points

1. Consumers should influence every stage of the research programme.
2. Those who give the care and those who receive it may have different perceptions of what constitutes good care.
3. Involving consumers in research helps in the identification of outcomes that are relevant and reliable.
4. Consumer involvement in audit ensures a clear focus on what matters to patients and clients.
5. It is rarely sufficient to involve just one consumer in research. She is unlikely to represent all the views of people using the service.
6. Consumers and health professionals working together on research need to clarify their respective roles, the outcomes to be measured and the extent to which it will be possible to incorporate results into practice.
7. Health professionals and consumers must respect each other's knowledge, skills and commitment to the research.
8. Both consumers and professionals need educating in how to work together.
9. It is important to evaluate the process of collaboration with consumers so that future research initiatives will be more effective.

and to find out what lessons can be learned for promoting future collaboration.

'Inevitably, attempts to reflect lay views in research will result in negative and positive experiences … It is therefore important that experiences from diverse settings are documented and made available for others to learn from.' (Entwistle et al 1998)

That collaboration is essential is not in question:

'It is only by acknowledging the views of women that maternity care will remain sensitive to changing social attitudes and greater empowerment of clients.' (Hall & Holloway 1998).

FURTHER READING

There are a number of seminal reports which explore the rationale behind involving consumers in research, detail how such involvement can be achieved and describe successful initiatives.

Joule N *User Involvement in Medical Audit* London: Greater London Association of Community Health Councils; 1992
This survey looks at the involvement of CHCs and users throughout the audit cycle. It can be obtained from The Greater London Association of Community Health Councils, 100 Park Village East, London, NW1 3SR, UK.

Kelson M *Consumer Involvement Initiatives in Clinical Audit and Outcomes* London: College of Health; 1995
The consumer sub-group of the Clinical Outcomes Group commissioned this Report through the College of Health to catalogue published literature on consumer involvement.

Oliver S, Buchanan P *Examples of Lay Involvement in Research and Development* London: EPI Centre; 1997
This Report explores lay perceptions of the NHS R&D programme and other health care research. It can be obtained from the EPI Centre, Social Science Research Unit, London University Institute of Education, 18 Woburn Square, London, WC1H 0NS, UK.

Fleming B, Golding L *Involving Users: Volume 1* Birmingham: Soundings Research; 1997
This booklet provides concise summaries of key concepts and methods in user involvement in health care. It can be obtained from Soundings Research, 377 Heath Road South, Northfield, Birmingham, B31 2BA, UK.

NHS Executive *Research: What's in it for Consumers?* London: Department of Health; 1997
This is the first Report of the Standing Advisory Group on Consumer Involvement in the NHS R&D Programme to the Central Research and Development Committee 1996/7.

REFERENCES

Chalmers I 'What do I want from health research and researchers when I am a patient?' *British Medical Journal* 1995; **310:** 1315–1318

Critical Appraisal Skills Programme: a multi-disciplinary approach Workshop One Oxford: Oxford Institute of Health Sciences; 1996

Department of Health *Consumers and Research in the NHS: Involving Consumers in Local Health Care* London: Department of Health; 1995

Enkin M, Keirse MJNC, Renfrew M, Neilson J *A Guide to Effective Care in Pregnancy and Childbirth* Second edition Oxford: Oxford University Press; 1995

Entwistle VA, Renfrew MJ, Yearley S, Forrester J, Lamont T 'Lay Perspectives: advantages for health research' *British Medical Journal* 1998; **316:** 463–466

Expert Maternity Group *Changing Childbirth* London: Department of Health; 1993

Fleming B, Golding L *Involving Users*, Volume 1. Birmingham: Soundings Research

Fletcher G, Buggins E, Newburn M, Gready M, Draper J, Wang M *The Voices Project: Training and Support for Maternity Services User Representatives* London: The National Childbirth Trust; 1997

Gready M, Newburn M, Dodds R, Gauge S *Birth Choices: Women's Expectations and Experiences* London: National Childbirth Trust; 1995

Gyte G 'Putting Research into Practice in Maternity Care' *Modern Midwife* 1994: 19–20

Hall SM, Holloway IM 'Staying in Control: women's experiences of labour in water' *Midwifery* 1998; **14(1):** 30–36

Hope I *The Use of Evidence-based Information for Enhancing Patient Choice* Report to the Anglia and Oxford Regional Health Authority; 1995

House of Commons *Second Report on the Maternity Services* (Winterton Report) London: HMSO; 1992

Joule N *User Involvement in Medical Audit* London: The Greater London Association of Community Health Councils; 1992

Kelson M *Consumer Involvement Initiatives in Clinical Audit and Outcomes* London: College of Health; 1995

LMCA (Long-Term Medical Conditions Alliance) *A New Partnership – Patients Influencing Purchasers* London: LMCA; (undated)

Matthews D 'User groups' *Changing Childbirth Update* 1998; **11**

Mays N, Pope C *Qualitative Research in Health Care* London: BMJ Publishing Group; 1996

Milne R 'Piloting Short Workshops on the Critical Appraisal of Reviews' *Health Trends* 1995; **27(4):** 120–123

NHS Centre for Reviews and Dissemination Report 7 *A Pilot Study of 'Informed Choice' Leaflets on Positions in Labour and Routine Ultrasound* London: Social Science Research Unit University of London Institute of Education; 1996

NHS Executive *Research: What's in it for Consumers?* First report of the Standing Advisory Group on Consumer Involvement in the NHS R&D Programme to the Central Research and Development Committee 1996/7 London: Department of Health; 1998

NHS Executive *Patient Partnerships* Birmingham: NHS Executive; 1997

Oliver S 'The Progress of Lay Involvement in the NHS Research and Development Programme' *Journal of Evaluation in Clinical Practice* 1996; **2(4):** 273–280

Oliver S, Buchanan P *Examples of Lay Involvement in Research & Development* London: London University Institute of Education EPI Centre; 1997

Proctor SR 'What Determines Quality in Maternity Care? Comparing the Perceptions of Childbearing Women and Midwives' *Birth* 1998; **25(2):** 85–93

Renfrew M, McCandlish R 'With Women: new steps in research in midwifery' in Roberts H *Women's Health Matters* London: Routledge; 1992

Smith CH, Armstrong D 'Comparison of Criteria Derived by Government and Patients From Evaluating General Practitioner Services.' *British Medical Journal* 1989; **299:** 494–496

6

Reviewing existing knowledge

Jennifer Hall and Sue Hawkins

KEY ISSUES

- Why do we need to review knowledge?
- How do we review knowledge?

- Where do we review knowledge?
- What do we do with that knowledge when we have found it?

INTRODUCTION

The chapter will explore issues involved in establishing what we need to know before we are able to address any research question. Other research books have generally called such a chapter 'Reviewing the literature'. However, it is important to realize that there are many *other* sources of knowledge in addition to the written word. The advent of technology has provided access to information by computer and many databases are now stored on CD-ROM. It is essential not to ignore other sources of information. Sources for discovering knowledge will be discussed. These include:

- colleagues
- libraries
- journals
- databases
- books.

Information will be provided about how to record the information and use it effectively. The chapter will conclude with a demonstration of critiquing a research report.

WHY REVIEW KNOWLEDGE?

> **Box 6.1** Reflection
>
> Before you read further spend a few minutes brainstorming the answer to this question: 'Why do we need to review knowledge?'

A simple answer could be that there is a need to establish what is already known or not known before setting out to answer a research question. If there is a great amount of knowledge available on a particular subject, you may find you can answer your question without going further. It may be necessary to change your proposed research project to one in which there is less knowledge or you may choose to replicate a particular study (Sleep 1985).

Reviews are used in different ways:

- as part of the research process to inform the researcher of the present knowledge on a subject and the methods used for previous research
- to provide information on issues of clinical relevance to influence practice and perhaps to provide a basis for standards
- as part of an academic course, which may be used as a source for future research projects (Rees 1997).

It is important to remember that '… any review of the evidence is only as good as the evidence that exists' (Renfrew 1997a). This implies that, if there are poor research studies on a particular issue, the review of these studies will be limited. However, a review can serve to identify weaknesses in studies and provide a stepping-stone for future research. Problems with reviewing knowledge are:

- finding all the relevant published and unpublished material
- assessing the quality of the studies identified (Renfrew 1997b).

The 'finding' part can be a long and arduous process, and it saves a lot of time if it is approached in a logical way.

HOW DO WE REVIEW KNOWLEDGE?

Subject matter

It is fundamental to a research project or review, to establish the *right question* in the first place. What do I want to find out? Why am I interested? What value would this study be to the profession? To the care of women and babies? As the questions are asked it may be appropriate to begin the search for answers by discussing them with colleagues. Talking around the subject may:

- help to focus the question on what is important
- establish alternative directions for the research
- feed into the review by offering appropriate sources of information.

It is important, before embarking on a review, to have a plan for its direction. It is very easy to be side-tracked once the search is under way. Searching the indexes or databases will reveal that a number of subjects may be listed together under a broader heading. Therefore, it is useful to create a list of key words that are appropriate to the subject of the research (Murphy-Black 1994). The principles of searching for key words are:

- use nouns
- include spelling variations; for example, the subject of breastfeeding may be recorded as breastfeeding, breastfeeding, or breast-feeding and caesarean may be spelt cesarean.
- include different terms for issues; for example, breastfeeding studies may be recorded under lactation.

Box 6.2   Key words

If you were preparing a review for the question 'Which midwives prefer working in teams?', what key words would you use?

In the above case, key words could be: team midwifery; case-loads; group practices; organizational change; midwives' roles; attitudes; satisfaction; continuity of care/carer; midwife led care; one-to-one care; named midwife. These are all words which could be used to describe aspects of this topic. As a secondary exploration, burn-out, stress and part-time occupational issues could also be explored.

Once key words have been established, sources of information need to be accessed.

WHERE TO REVIEW KNOWLEDGE?

The last few years have seen a rapid growth in the amount of information being published and made available to midwives. In 1983 when MIDIRS (Midwives Information and Resource Service) was set up, many midwives had little access to information of any sort. Now there are over half a dozen midwifery journals in the UK alone and new databases spring up at an exciting rate. We have witnessed huge changes in technology and the development of the Internet has opened up access to information in a way that has both delighted and frustrated those of us trying to find relevant, authoritative and timely information.

Libraries

University and hospital libraries are key places to find information. However, for each library you use, it is important:

- to know what is available in terms of subject matter, journals, indexes, databases, and facilities
- to know if there is a system for booking the use of the databases or computer terminals

- to know what can be ordered from other sources, locally and nationally
- to know the costs of ordering, photocopying, printing and other facilities
- to establish positive links with the librarian who can be a valuable source of information.

It can be very frustrating to travel to a library and then discover that it is not the correct one for the subject to be studied. Equally, it can be upsetting to realize that the database terminals are pre-booked for the time you have available. The knowledge of cost is important, as it is vital to keep expense to a minimum: if another library has the same facilities but cheaper photocopying, then it may be more appropriate to go there. For the researcher, time is valuable and being informed saves time.

Sources

Journals

Printed journals are still the main forum for the publication of research papers and they allow health professionals to keep up to date with new research and to share their experiences of practice. Journals offer a convenient, easy-to-read format for the publication of research and are generally the fastest way of disseminating new research to a large number of people. However, it is worth noting that the delay between completion of research and publication can still be considerable.

When reading journal articles it is important to establish whether or not the journal is peer reviewed. Until recently there were few, if any, well researched and peer reviewed journals on the market for midwives in Britain. The situation has improved, but midwives will need to look at key obstetric and general medical journals as well. The journals listed in Table 6.1 are only a few of the hundreds of titles covering midwifery, obstetrics and general medicine but have been chosen as the most useful for midwives.

Databases

There are a number of databases available now which are applicable and accessible to midwives. These may be accessed through libraries, as suggested, though some are now available as subscriptions, on CD-ROM, or on the Internet. Most are also produced in the printed form. Some are easier to use than others and the librarian can be helpful in providing guidance. Be aware, too, that they may not carry all the information that is required, if there has been inaccurate indexing or if the authors have failed to provide correct information (Shennan & Shennan 1996). Table 6.2 provides a summary of some of the databases that are available and useful to midwives. Many more are being developed and librarians will be able

Table 6.1 Some of the most useful journals for midwives

Title	Features	Contact details
Midwifery	• Essential reading: research articles; of central relevance to midwifery. • Articles are refereed and of a very high standard. • Published quarterly.	Harcourt Brace & Co Ltd, Foots Cray, Sidcup, Kent, England DA14 5HP. http://www.churchillmed.com/Midwifery/jhome.html
British Journal of Midwifery	• Essential reading original research which is peer reviewed and refereed. • Some articles are available on the Mark Allen web site. • Published monthly.	Mark Allen Publishing, Croxted Mews, 288 Croxted Road, London, SE24 9BY. http://www.MarkAllenGroup.com/bjm.htm
The Practising Midwife	• New journal combines anecdotal features and articles based on research evidence. • Some original research, anonymous peer reviews. • Useful feature – Cochrane made simple series – where editors provide a summary of Cochrane reviews. • Published quarterly.	Hochland & Hochland, 174a Ashley Road, Hale, Cheshire, England, WA15 9SE.
Birth	• Recommended reading; articles of highest standard; well referenced and accurate. • All articles are refereed. • Published quarterly.	Blackwell Scientific Publications, Commerce Place, 350 Main Street, Malden, Massachusetts, USA. http://www.blackwell-science.com
Journal of Nurse Midwifery	• Official publication of American College of Nurse-Midwives. • Articles of variable quality, but generally one or two of interest in each issue. • Published bi-monthly.	Elsevier Science Inc. 655 Avenue of the Americas, New York, NY10010, USA. http://www.elsevier.nl/inca/publications/store/5/0/5/7/7/4/
British Journal of Obstetrics and Gynaecology	• Official journal of Royal College of Obstetricians and Gynaecologists. • Important journal. • Obstetric articles often highly relevant to midwives. • Articles are refereed and standard is generally high. • Published monthly.	Subscription information from: Journal Customer services; Blackwell Scientific Publications Ltd, Osney Mead, Oxford, OX2 0EL. http://www.blackwell-science.com

Table 6.1 *(contd)*

Title	Features	Contact details
British Medical Journal	• Journal of the British Medical Association. • Only a few articles will be relevant to midwifery, but these will be of central importance. • All articles are refereed and of the highest standard. • Published weekly.	BMJ, BMA House, Tavistock Square, London, WC1H 9TD. http://www.bmj.com
The Lancet	• Only a few articles will probably be relevant to midwives, but these will be of central importance. • All articles are refereed and of the highest standard. • Published weekly.	The Lancet, 46 Bedford Square, London, WC1B 3SL. http://www.thelancet.com
Evidence-Based Medicine	• From over 70 journals, key research papers are presented in a structured abstract with reviewer's comments. • Includes specialties of obstetrics and paediatrics and has papers of relevance to midwives.	Specialist Journals Dept. BMJ Publishing Group, BMA House, Tavistock Square, London. http://www.bmjpg.com/data/ebmb.htm
Evidence-Based Nursing	• Review journal as above. • First published Jan 1998, and has included at least 12 articles of relevance to midwives.	As above. http://www.evidencebasednursing.com

Table 6.2 Databases for research in midwifery

Database	Format	Content	Benefits (B) and Limitations (L)
Cochrane Library: • Cochrane database of systematic reviews (CDSR)	CD-ROM	Systematic reviews of randomized controlled trials.	B: full text, information collated and compared, meta-analysis, editing and reviewing by number of people and disciplines, giving accurate information. Used by practitioners to inform and change practice. L: some complaints about ease of use, expense and access to information.
• NHS Centre for Reviews and Dissemination (CRD) database of abstracts of reviews of effectiveness (DARE)		• Abstracts of systematic reviews assessed by CRD • Abstracts of reviews from American College of Physicians Journal Club • International network of Agencies for Health Technology Assessments • Refs for review articles that do not meet CRD criteria but have been assessed • Refs for review articles that have not been assessed.	
• Cochrane Controlled Trials Register • Cochrane review methodology database		Refs of controlled trials. Refs to books, journals articles on methodology, of trials, systematic reviews and meta-analysis.	
MIDIRS midwifery database	Sourced through MIDIRS (may be soon on CD-ROM or on-line) via telephone, fax or website, Midwifery Digest.	Over 60 000 refs hand-searched from over 550 journals, consumer magazines, self-help newsletters, newspaper articles, government publications. All articles abstracted.	B: bibliographic database specifically for midwives, saves time on library journeys, can access information quickly, can obtain photocopies of obscure journals from MIDIRS. L: need to be specific with key words, photocopies expensive, sometimes slow to obtain information.

Table 6.2 *(contd)*

Database	Format	Content	Benefits (B) and Limitations (L)
MIRIAD	Sourcebook	Ongoing and completed research including aims, design data collection, sampling, analysis, results, publications.	B: source of information on ongoing studies. Specific to midwives. Book format may make it accessible to all but also limits it as well.
MEDLINE	CD-ROM, on-line, Index Medicus	Scans + 3700 biomedical journals. Abstracts available if author abstract given.	B: volume of data. L: American and medical slant – keywords may be different. No books, reports or consumer literature. Dependent on author information.
CINAHL (Cumulative Index to Nursing and Allied Health Literature)	CD-ROM, printed, on-line	1000 journals nursing, midwifery, other health specialities.	B: focused on nursing and midwifery issues. L: American slant.
BNI (British Nursing Index)	CD-ROM, printed, University of Bournemouth website	220 journals nursing, midwifery, health visitors and others. Nursing and Midwifery index from 1994, RCN nursing bibliography from 1995, and RCN CD-ROM 115 000 + records.	B: focused on nursing and midwifery issues. L: no abstracts.
ASSIA (Applied Social Sciences Index and Abstracts)	CD-ROM, Index	Reviews, English language journals, sociology, psychology and health.	B: useful for information relating to psychology and sociology. L: limited to specific journals.
ENB Health care	CD-ROM, ENB website	25 000 records from 60 journals, open learning packs, and information about organizations. For educators, managers and clinicians.	B: specific information for midwives, wide range of material. L: few journals, lack of accessibility.

Table 6.2 (contd)

Database	Format	Content	Benefits (B) and Limitations (L)
HMIC:			
• Kings Fund library	CD-ROM	260 000 records from 1983, books, pamphlets, journal articles on NHS management, development and organization, GP funding and healthcare financing.	B: focused on health management, wide range of material. L: limited accessibility.
• DOH database		Health service administration, equipment and supplies, social services, primary care and public health.	
• Nuffield list of health		54 000 refs to articles, books, reports on health systems in UK, Europe and developed countries.	
RCM	Computer-based catalogue	Catalogue of books and reports in RCM library.	B: midwifery focused, books can be borrowed from a distance. L: only available to RCM members, database only accessible in RCM library, though telephone orders may be taken.
National Research Register (NRR) • Register of registers	CD-ROM, plans for Internet or NHSnet	Ongoing NHS research funded by NHS R&D levy – 6000 projects. Information on other registers with similar R&D project info.	B: useful for current research. L: limited accessibility but plans for CD-ROM and access via NHSnet; limited quality control.
• MRC Clinical Trials Directory • NHS CRD reviews in progress register		Information about clinical trials in receipt of MRC grants, in total + 20–30 000 records.	
National Clinical Audit Database	From RCOG Clinical Audit Unit	Information about audit in maternity care and gynaecology, over 5000 records.	B: relevant to midwives, information available free.
Maternity Practice Database	From RCOG Clinical Audit Unit	Information on research, projects, initiatives of good practice in relation to maternity care, about 495 entries.	B: relevant to midwives, information free. L: limited accessibility.

to give information on what is available locally. Databases *particularly* relevant to midwives are

- the Cochrane library
- MIDIRS
- MIRIAD
- National Clinical Audit Database
- Maternity Practice Database
- the RCM
- the National Research Register.

The Cochrane Library. The information in the Cochrane Library is valuable to midwives. For instance the Cochrane Database of Systematic Reviews (CDSR) carries all the information on randomized, controlled trials of a subject, which has been collated, compared and then synthesized to produce an overall summary. Editing and reviewing of the data has been undertaken by a number of people from different disciplines and countries (Renfrew 1997b). This has ensured that the information is as correct as possible. The process of review and synthesis is called *meta-analysis*, and it has enabled clinicians to use the information confidently as a basis for changing practice. The current version of the database (1998, Issue 3) contains 428 systematic reviews, of which over 180 are directly relevant to midwives. There have been some concerns about access and availability of the information (Meah et al 1996), so some trusts have developed workbooks to use alongside the database as a learning tool (Alexander et al 1996).

The Cochrane Pregnancy and Childbirth Database (CCPC) is no longer available. A programme of updating these reviews to the Cochrane format for addition to CDSR is currently under way.

The Cochrane Library also has information about the approximately 50 review groups that have been set up, including the Pregnancy and Childbirth Review Group and the Neonatal Review Group.

The Cochrane Controlled Trials Register is a collection of references to controlled trials in health care. These have been identified by the Cochrane Collaboration Groups by hand-searching journals, and this has highlighted studies which were not available on other electronic databases. A quick search using terms to identify articles using these key words: pregnancy; labour; postnatal; midwifery; newborn, yielded over 12 000 references.

It is worth looking at the Cochrane web site (www.cochrane.co.uk) as this provides information about the initiative and also gives access to the abstracts of the reviews, which are arranged within review groups.

MIDIRS Midwifery database. This is one of the most useful databases for midwives. MIDIRS is a charitable organization supporting a database of over 60 000 sources. This includes lay material, and government papers, as well as medical, nursing and midwifery journals. Most of the references are from 1985 onwards, but there are almost 2000 earlier references, the oldest being 1857.

There are over 350 lists of references based on the most popular enquiries received from midwives. These lists are updated every month and can be supplied by post, fax or e-mail. There are plans to make these lists available on the MIDIRS website so they can be printed off locally by anyone using the website. If the subject required is not one covered by these lists, the information staff can search the database for references on any subject on request. In 1997 over 20 000 subject enquiries were answered in this way. There are plans to make the database more widely available on CD-ROM or via the Internet.

Advantages to using MIDIRS are:

- queries can be dealt with over the telephone
- you do not have to spend a long time in a library on a search
- the information is pertinent to midwives
- the material may be accessed afterwards through the photocopying service. Bear in mind that the photocopying service is quite expensive and this should to be weighed up with the time saved through the search being performed for you.

Whilst all relevant articles are added to the MIDIRS Midwifery database, those that are methodologically sound and of prime relevance to midwives are selected for inclusion in the MIDIRS Midwifery Digest. These are usually stocked in libraries, and are recognizable by their bright pink colour (Hawkins 1998). Articles are sent to experts in the field for review or comment. Commentaries take the form of a lengthy review on the original paper and may include the original author abstract. Since its inception, over 1000 research studies have been abstracted in this way.

MIRIAD. This database originated at the National Perinatal Epidemiology unit in Oxford, run by the Midwifery Research Programme and funded by the Department of Health. Started in 1988, it is a collection of United Kingdom midwifery research studies on a computerized database. Since 1995 it has been run from the Department of Midwifery Studies (now the Mother and Infant Research Unit) at the University of Leeds. It was published regularly in book form, the fifth report (the third one published by Books for Midwives Press) published in 1997. The database contains over 400 research studies relating to clinical, management, historical or educational issues. The book presents details of the studies as prepared and submitted by the authors. It is useful in that it contains summaries of studies that have never been published or that are still to be completed. The accessibility is via the source book or through telephoning the department. But books take time to be published and more recent studies may not be included in the current edition. Also, there is no analysis of the quality or value of the studies, leaving the reader to critique the information.

Each study has a list of keywords and there is a keyword index, which is useful for searching this and other sources for research information. The database was funded by the National Research Register (NRR) until March 1999. The NRR now maintain the information. There are plans to publish the database on the Internet.

Royal College of Midwives (RCM). The recent move of the RCM library to larger premises has provided the means for development of a computerized database of the contents of the library. At present it does not include the contents of journals. It is available by appointment during office hours through visiting the RCM premises in London. Information may also be obtained through telephoning. A search may be performed for you for a minimal charge. A postal loan service is also available to RCM members, with the borrower paying postage. A limited photocopying service is available, though written application should be made and orders are limited to six.

National Clinical Audit and Maternity Practice Databases. These databases were developed and maintained by the RCOG Clinical Audit Unit in Manchester from 1991 to 1999. In May 1999 they were relocated to the RCOG in London where they are currently available. The National Clinical Audit database contains over 5000 audit initiatives relating to maternity care and gynaecology. The Maternity Practice database was previously known as the Changing Childbirth Contacts Register. It contains information on research and projects in relation to maternity care and includes unpublished projects. Books and leaflets, lists of organizations and initiatives of good practice are also included. Contact names and addresses are available for the projects concerned. Entries are recorded through key words and each includes an abstract. Access to the information is through direct contact with the RCOG, and provision of the information is, at present, a free service.

National Research Register. This database contains information on research funded directly by the NHS, or through the NHS R&D programme (see Chapter 3). The aims of the database are to support efficient research management and reduce duplication, commissioning of new research, assessing money spent on research and to give input to research overviews. Access to the database is through R&D managers within regional offices of the NHS Executive. There are, however, plans to make the database available via the Internet or NHSnet in the future. At present, there are problems accessing the database easily and, as a result of the large number of projects included (more than 40 000), there are problems of quality control of the information.

British Nursing Index. This has developed as a result of collaboration between the Royal College of Nursing Library and the Nursing and Midwifery Index Consortium of Libraries. Articles indexed are those likely to be of interest to nurses, midwives, health visitors and allied professionals.

The BNI can be accessed on CD-ROM or through the University of Bournemouth website (registration required). It is most likely to be of interest to midwives when used as an adjunct to midwifery databases such as MIDIRS. Many of the clinical research articles available on BNI will be available through CINAHL or MEDLINE, or, if on midwifery, through the MIDIRS Midwifery database. The main strength of BNI is that it is British in origin. This means that topics such as Primary Care Groups, the National Health Service and other subjects unique to the UK are well covered. Another advantage is that many of the journals cited will be widely available in health care libraries.

These are just a few of the databases of interest to midwives. There are many others which may be of use, and readers are urged to consult their librarians for advice on the most relevant. Two useful sources are found in Carmel (1995), which has a chapter on computerized literature searching, and Carmel and Sawers (1996), which gives details of over 280 databases produced by medical libraries, public libraries and voluntary organizations.

When searching databases for information it is helpful to remember:

- One database is unlikely to have all the information required.
- Indexes are often available if the CD-ROM is in use.
- The process of searching takes time.

Accessing research reports

The process of searching the databases, as described, should provide a list of relevant references and abstracts. The next steps in the process, prior to searching the shelves, are given below:

1. Read through the list of references and attempt to assess the usefulness of the report from the abstract provided. Does the title suggest it is relevant to the research question? Is it a report of a research study, or a review or discussion paper?

2. Prioritize the search for papers according to perceived journal quality. Those that are peer-reviewed tend to carry more weight. However, do not completely discount other journals, especially if the intended study is more descriptive or qualitative in nature.

3. Does your local library hold the journals? Begin with those journals that are stocked. Order other articles from the British Library (some libraries may limit the number that may be ordered, also beware of the cost), or try MIDIRS.

4. Particular journals may be more relevant, such as, midwifery-based journals or specialist journals such as the *Journal of Human Lactation*, or *Journal of Perinatal and Neonatal Nursing*. Therefore, consider accessing an index from these journals (some may not have them) or hand search back

3 to 5 years to see if there are other appropriate studies. This process takes time and beware of being side-tracked.

5. On finding a study, quickly scan read it to assess if it is relevant. Do not photocopy everything as it is expensive. Do cross a paper off the list if it is not appropriate, or you could waste time searching for it again.

6. Remember that papers generally have references at the end. These can be used to search for further useful papers.

Books

It goes without saying that libraries contain books! However, it is important to remember that a particular library may not contain the subject required nor will it contain all the books written on a particular subject. Therefore, as indicated at the beginning, it is worth finding out what each library holds before making a visit that may waste time.

When the right library has been accessed there are two ways of discovering appropriate titles:

1. Use the library computer database to search for a subject.
2. Find the area that holds the subject required and hand-search the shelves.

The first method will ensure that you obtain a list of appropriate titles and will indicate if they are situated in a different library or out on loan. The second method may mean that you discover titles that you would not have identified via the database, because of the problem of using correct key words. Both methods are equally valid and useful.

However, it should be remembered that books take months or years to write and be published. Therefore, more recent research papers may replace the information on which a book is based. It is necessary to assess the information very carefully.

Other sources

There are other sources of research information that may be accessed by midwives.

- Individual projects such as MSc studies or PhD studies. These are held in the British Library and the library of the awarding university.
- Organizational projects including Government research, institutional research, such as drug or infant formula companies, or charitable organizations, and research instituted by organizations such as the UKCC or RCM. These may be accessed via the inter-library loan service in universities, through the RCM library, the British Library or through the individual or organization concerned. Be prepared to use the telephone

to track down reports. The MIRIAD books are particularly useful in providing this information.

The process of finding information takes time and patience. The search may produce a lot of material, in which case the research question may need to be limited or made more specific. If it produces only a limited amount, the topic may need to be broadened. The next phase is to extract the relevant information.

ASSESSING AND RECORDING INFORMATION

The next step in the process is to assess the research material, and then to store it ready to write the review. A set of themes should be created that will form the basis for the review. It is advisable to begin by skim reading each paper and assessing its relevance. When the best have been selected, they should be read in more detail and the information recorded. There are different ways of doing this. Try:

• highlighter pens
• index card system
• grid system
• computer.

Table 6.3 provides a summary of how these may be used and lists advantages and disadvantages for each method. As a researcher, it is advisable to use a method that you find easy to use, but that will also be fast. Use of a computer may be appropriate, but not if it is going to take a lot of time trying to understand unfamiliar programs or if it is going to be frequently inaccessible. It is important to weigh up which is the most appropriate for you.

EVALUATING RESEARCH

The review, when written, will not be just a collection of descriptions of research articles, but should include critical analysis. This involves making judgements about the process of research, the validity of the results and the appropriateness of the conclusions drawn in each case. The process will be slightly different for quantitative and qualitative papers. Scientific research papers are generally presented using particular formats and headings:

• *Title* – provides a key to the theme or focus of the study.
• *Abstract* – a summary of the study in about 200 words, providing key points on how the research was carried out and conclusions drawn.
• *Introduction* – demonstrates the background and says why the researcher carried out the study.

Table 6.3 Recording information

Method	Advantages	Disadvantages
Highlighter pens – read through articles and highlight different subjects in different colours.	Cheap, quick to use.	Some papers will be covered in lines making it hard to compare at the writing stage. Makes photocopying difficult. Easy to lose.
Index cards – use one or two sets of different colours. One has the complete reference written, and is kept in alphabetical order of author. The other carries an appropriate quote for subject with author's name as a cross-reference.	Cheap, easy to access information. May be laid out in order of use at writing stage.	Takes time to write out information. Easy to lose.
Grid – consists of large piece of paper divided into columns. Each column represents a theme of the review. Rees (1997) suggests labelling them: • Terms of reference/hypothesis • Research design/method of data collection.	Cheap. Ease of comparison between research articles. Highlights similarities and differences. Useful for giving an overview of a review especially for higher degree work.	Time to write it out initially.
Computer – Rees (1997) suggests the following: • Create a file for each theme. • Place information from research article into each file. • Start each quotation with name of author, year of publication and page number.	If using a word processing package it is easy to move quotes around and add them to the review as it is being written.	Need to have access to computer and knowledge of use. May lose the information if an error is made.
Reference managers such as Procite, Endnote Plus, Reference Manager, Papyrus.	Best for handling large numbers of references. Can be used to organize all bibliographic information: explore which is the best program for your type of use. When writing up program can modify for different reference styles, eg. Vancouver or Harvard.	Need some practice with managing a database. Not the cheapest option financially. Need back up copies to protect.

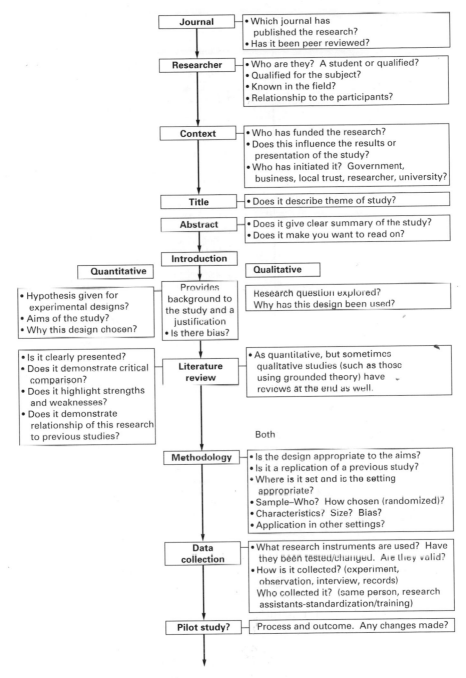

Figure 6.1 Critical analysis pathway

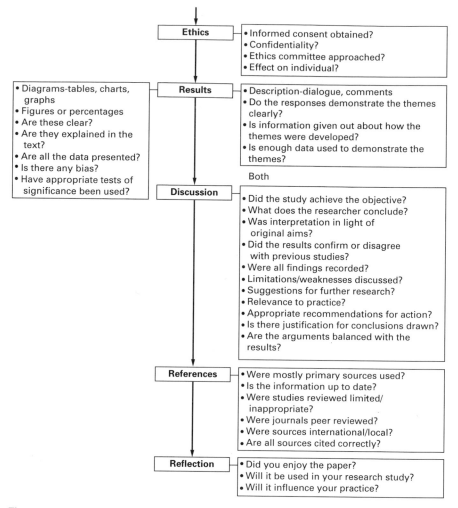

Figure 6.1b   (contd)

- *Review of the literature* – demonstrates critical appraisal, building on previous research, knowledge of the field.
- *The research question* – for quantitative experimental studies an hypothesis should also be stated.
- *Method* – a description of how the study was carried out.
- *Results* – the result of the study and an interpretation.
- *Discussion* – a critical analysis of the results and comparison with previous studies. May include recommendations, limitations and implications for practice.

- *Conclusion* – summary of the study.
- *References* – a complete list of all the papers referred to within the paper.

Qualitative studies may be similar, but some may have the literature review included in the discussion at the end to ensure the findings are grounded in the data (Clark 1991).

Figure 6.1 illustrates a pathway of critical analysis with questions that may be asked when critiquing a paper. These questions can be asked when critically reading any research and may enable the reader to assess effectively the quality of the work.

CONCLUSION

Prior to starting any research study it is appropriate and valuable to examine the information that is already available on a subject. This chapter has listed available sources of this information for midwives and demonstrated how this information may be accessed and recorded. A pathway of how to analyse research papers critically is described. Within this context it is useful to reiterate that the process of finding information is a logical progression and that the process takes time if it is to be done well.

FURTHER READING

Anthony D Midwives on the Internet *British Journal of Midwifery* 1996; 4(12): 645–648
Describes the resources available on the Internet for Midwives. Also suggests future developments for midwifery usage.
Bowles N Using the Internet to Support Midwifery Practice *British Journal of Midwifery* 1996; 4(12): 649–652
Another article providing a beginner's guide to use of the Internet with resources available for midwives.
Nursing Times & NHS Executive *Clinical Effectiveness for Nurses, Midwives and Health Visitors*. London: EMAP Healthcare; 1998
A publication that summarizes the process of development of clinical effectiveness. Contains a basic chapter on searching the literature with other useful references.

REFERENCES

Alexander J, Gwyer R, Pitman B 'Collaborating on Cochrane and Disseminating the Database' *British Journal of Midwifery* 1996; **4(12)**: 637–639
Carmel M *Health Care Librarianship and Information Work* Second edition London: Library Association Publishing; 1995
Carmel S, Sawers C *Directory of Health and Social Services Database* based on research funded by the British Library Research and Development Department. London: Library Association Publishing; 1996
Clark E *Evaluating research Module 10* London: Distance Learning Centre, South Bank Polytechnic; 1991
Hawkins S 'Finding the Evidence: a guide to information sources in midwifery' *British Journal of Midwifery* 1998; **6(4)**: 215–219
Meah S, Luker KA, Cullum NA 'An Exploration of Midwives' Attitudes to Research and

Perceived Barriers to Research Utilisation' *Midwifery* 1996; **12:** 73–84

Murphy-Black T 'Searching the Midwifery Literature' *British Journal of Midwifery* 1994; **2(9):** 441–443

Rees C *An Introduction to Research for Midwives* Hale, Cheshire: Books for Midwives Press; 1997

Renfrew MJ 'The Development of Evidence-based Practice' *British Journal of Midwifery* 1997a; **5(2):** 100–104

Renfrew MJ 'Influencing the Development of Evidence-based Practice '*British Journal of Midwifery* 1997b; **5(3):** 131–132, 134

Shennan C, Shennan A 'The Cochrane Database: the way ahead' *British Journal of Midwifery* 1996; **4(12):** 640–644

Sleep J 'Things I Wish I'd Known Before I Started' *Midwifery* 1985; **(1):** 54–57

Guides to sources on the Internet

Anthony D 'Midwives on the Internet' *British Journal of Midwifery* 1996; **4(12):** 645–648

Bowles N 'Using the Internet to Support Midwifery Practice' *British Journal of Midwifery* 1996; **4(12):** 649–652

Kiley R *Medical Information on the Internet: a guide for health professionals* Edinburgh: Churchill Livingstone; 1996

Sinclair M 'Midwives, Midwifery and the Internet' *Modern Midwife* 1997; **7(9):** 11–14

Resources

British Library
Thorp Arch Trading Estate
Boston Spa, North Yorkshire
England
Tel: 01937 546060

BNI Publications
Library and Information Services
Bournemouth University
Dorset House, Talbot Campus
Fern Barrow, Poole, Dorset,
BH12 5BB
Tel: 01201 595454
http://www.bni.org.uk/cgi-bin/index.html

CINAHL – http://www.cinahl.com

The Cochrane Library
The Cochrane Collaboration
BMJ Publishing Group
PO Box 295
London
WC1H 9TE
Tel: 0171 383 6185/6245
http://www.cochrane.org.uk

English National Board
Victory House
170 Tottenham Court Road
London
W1P 0HA
Tel: 0171 391 6260
http://www.enb.org.uk

MEDLINE http://www.nlm.gov/databases/freemedl.htm

MIDIRS
9 Elmdale Road
Clifton
Bristol BS8 1SL
Tel: 0117 925 1791
http://www.midirs.org

MIRIAD
Mother and Infant Research Unit
University of Leeds
22 Hyde Terrace
Leeds
LS2 9LN
Tel: 0113 233 6888
Email: f.m.mccormick@leeds.ac.uk

National Research Register
NHS Executive Headquarters RD3
Quarry House
Room GW59
Leeds
LS2 7UE

Optology Ltd. (publish HMIC)
Notition House
Menzies Road
St-Leonards-On-Sea
East Sussex
TN38 9BB
Tel: 01424 445100

Royal College of Midwives
15 Mansfield Street
London
W1M 0BE
Tel: 0171 872 5100
http://www.midwives.co.uk

Royal College of Nursing
20 Cavendish Square
London
W1M 0AB
Tel: 0171 409 3333

RCOG Clinical Audit Unit
St Mary's Hospital
Hathersage Road
Manchester
M13 0JH
Tel: 0161 276 6300
Email: audit@rcog.cmht.nwest.uk

7

Asking questions about practice and using appropriate research methods

Debra Bick

KEY ISSUES

- Research questions must be clearly defined. Many of the stages in the research process will be influenced by the nature of the question asked
- Research methods fall broadly into two complementary categories – qualitative or quantitative
- Some studies use a combination of methods, often referred to as 'triangulated' or 'multiple' methods

- It is important to consider at each stage of the research process if advice or assistance should be sought. Multi-disciplinary research is particularly important
- Reflective exercises at the end of each section will enable the prospective researcher to consider various issues before deciding if a particular research method is appropriate to answer their question.

INTRODUCTION

This is an exciting time for research in midwifery. Government reports on the maternity services (House of Commons Select Committee Report 1992, Department of Health 1993) have provided the impetus for a midwifery-led service, but if this is to be effective, practice must be based on evidence from rigorously conducted research. This chapter describes some of the questions which could be asked about practice and the appropriate research methods which could be used to answer them. Examples of relevant studies are given and the importance of using the expertise and skills of other professionals to strengthen research in midwifery are discussed.

ASKING QUESTIONS ABOUT PRACTICE

Questions can be influenced by many factors, such as an alteration to the pattern of care, concern about an aspect of practice, the need to evaluate new developments in practice, or from searching the literature. The following are a few examples of the sorts of questions that could be asked about practice (you will probably be able to think of many others):

- What factors influence the number of postnatal home visits made?
- What contribution will advanced midwifery practitioners make to the profession?
- What choices do women have about where to give birth?
- How can breastfeeding rates be improved?
- What are midwives' views of the impact of *Changing Childbirth* on their practice?

It is very important, before deciding which research method is appropriate, that the question is clearly defined and can be answered through the collection and analysis of data. This is a crucial part of the research process (see Figure 7.1). Many of the stages in the research process will be influenced by the nature of the question asked.

Practical issues should also be considered. These include the individual's previous research experience, financial costs of printing research instruments, postage, telephone calls, travel and the time required to complete a study, particularly if it is being undertaken in addition to a clinical role.

USING THE SKILLS AND EXPERTISE OF OTHER PROFESSIONALS

No prospective researcher, whatever their level of expertise, should feel that they have to go it alone when designing and undertaking research. Asking for advice and assistance is invaluable. It could prevent mistakes being made that would affect the outcome of the study and the motivation of the individual to do further research. Establishing links with other professionals is also a useful way of finding out about research they have undertaken or have access to, which could inform evidence-based practice. Professionals who could assist midwifery researchers include:

- social scientists
- psychologists
- health economists
- statisticians
- epidemiologists
- nurses
- obstetricians
- general practitioners.

Multi-disciplinary research is discussed in Chapter 3.

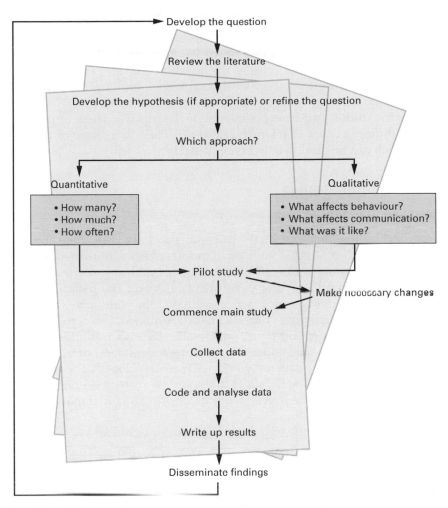

Figure 7.1   The research process

USING APPROPRIATE RESEARCH METHODS

Rees (1997) suggests that the decision regarding which method to use should be considered using the 'terms of reference'. This means that if the research question aims to ascertain women's views, opinions or experiences of the maternity services, methods designed to ascertain their views would be appropriate. If the research question is to find out how midwives interact with women in labour, observation would be appropriate. If the research question is to assess the effect of an alteration to midwifery practice, an experimental study would be appropriate. Many studies use a combination of methods, sometimes referred to as *triangulated* or *multiple methods*.

We now go on to consider different research methods and their suitability for different research questions. Examples of studies which have used each research method described are also given. These published studies have been selected because the question and the research method used to answer the question are clearly explained, and it is recommended that you read them.

Research studies can be experimental or descriptive. These approaches answer different types of research questions. There is a range of research tools which can be used in either type of study.

Experimental studies

Randomized controlled trials

Experimental research enables the researcher to state with some accuracy that one thing has affected another. Randomized controlled trials (RCT) are one of the most commonly used experimental approaches and are sometimes referred to as 'true experiments'. One of the most important RCTs to influence midwifery practice evaluated the routine use of episiotomy where the delivery was expected to be spontaneous (Sleep et al 1984). Prior to this trial there had been considerable dispute, but little scientific evidence concerning the short-term and long-term effects of episiotomy. Restrictive and liberal episiotomy policies were developed. The restrictive policy was defined as one in which the midwife restricted episiotomy to fetal indications only; the liberal policy as one in which the midwife tried to prevent a perineal tear.

Important questions the trial sought to answer included:

- Was there a higher incidence of perineal pain at 10 days and 3 months between the two groups?
- Was there a difference in the incidence of urinary incontinence at 3 months between the two groups?

The findings that there were no differences in perineal pain or urinary incontinence at 3 months suggested that there was little evidence to justify the routine use of episiotomy.

There are several reasons why RCTs are considered to be the 'gold standard' of research methods:

- Individuals are randomly allocated so that each has the same chance of receiving the intervention.
- Study groups tend to be similar with respect to all variables except for the intervention being studied.
- An RCT offers more conclusive evidence that the independent variable (e.g. a new package of midwifery care) has an effect on the dependent variable (e.g. prolonged duration of breastfeeding).

If treatments are not randomly allocated, bias cannot be ruled out as an explanation for apparent differences. Randomization can provide a degree of reassurance about the comparability of the study groups that is not possible in any other study design (Hennekins & Buring 1987).

It is important to note that although an RCT has been carried out, this does not necessarily mean that the study findings are valid. There may have been confounding factors where something outside of the study affected the outcome, or potential bias if the control group received *part* of the intervention being examined. Due to these difficulties, anyone contemplating an RCT should seek advice from experienced researchers in this method (including a statistician) and carefully read reports of published RCTs.

Non-random methods

It is not always possible, practically or ethically, to use a 'true experiment' and other ways of obtaining quantitative data have to be used. Non-random methods can be used, which are sometimes referred to as *quasi-experiments*. This means that although there has been an experimental and a control group, there has not been random allocation to the groups. Ex-post facto ('after the fact') refers to a study design where the participants are questioned after exposure to a particular event and are compared with a group who were not exposed to the same event.

Box 7.1   Is an experimental study the most appropriate method?

- Is the aim of your research to examine a cause and effect relationship?
- What are the main outcomes of your study and how will you collect data on these?
- Have you thought of any potential confounding factors which could bias the outcome of your study?
- Have you considered whether ethical problems could arise if the intervention is withheld from the control group?
- How will you ensure that the study participants adhere to the study protocol?
- How will you randomize your study participants?
- How will you collect, code and analyse the data?

Table 7.1   Examples of studies which have used experiments

Authors	Aim of study	Tools used
Rogers et al (1998)	To test the hypothesis that active management of the third stage of labour lowers the rate of primary postpartum haemorrhage.	Questionnaires, obstetric case note review.
Turnbull et al (1996)	To compare the clinical efficacy of and women's satisfaction with midwifery care and shared care.	Interviews, questionnaires, records of observations, obstetric case note review.

Descriptive studies

Descriptive studies set out simply to describe what exists; they cannot test cause and effect relationships. Such studies include, for example, *ethnography, case studies* and *surveys*. The survey is the most commonly used approach.

Surveys

A survey is a method of gathering data from a large number of people by directly asking them for information, and can collect qualitative and quantitative data. Surveys are described by Burnard & Morrison (1994) as 'a systematic gathering of information from a reasonably large sample of people, events, literature, records and so forth. The purpose of a survey is usually to identify general trends or patterns in data'.

Cartwright (1988) described surveys as a research tool which could be used to ascertain facts, confirm or refute theories, explore ideas and identify values. In health research, surveys are usually directed to answer more than one question. For example, if the research question was 'Do women who attend parentcraft classes cope better with labour pain than women who do not attend?', supplementary questions should be asked to find out 'which women coped better?' and 'in what way did they cope?'

Surveys can be *structured*, which means that the same questions are asked of all participants, or they can be *unstructured*, for example asking women for their views of what helped them to cope with pain during labour. A survey can be *cross-sectional* if it is used to obtain information about a specific event at one point in time, or *longitudinal* if subjects are followed up at several points in time to assess how changes have affected them. Questionnaires or interviews are generally used to collect data for a survey. A large national survey of women's views and experiences of the maternity services was carried out recently as part of a study by the Audit Commission (Garcia et al 1998) and one of the main findings was that women were dissatisfied with their postnatal care. The inclusion of questions to allow women to express their views highlighted the need for further research into this important area.

Box 7.2 Is a survey is the most appropriate method?

- Would a cross-sectional or longitudinal survey be more appropriate for your study?
- Do you have financial resources available to pay for any printing or postage costs?
- Are you confident that a survey will provide you with sufficiently detailed data?
- How will you collect, code and analyze the data?

Table 7.2   Example of a survey

Authors	Aim of study	How was the survey carried out?
Garcia et al (1998) A national survey of the maternity services carried out by the Audit Commission.	To obtain women's views and experiences of the maternity services.	Questionnaire

Case study

In a case study the researcher attempts to critically analyse and understand the factors that contributed to the history of an individual's problems or care. A number of tools can be used to collect information, including case review and interview data. A case study could be used, for example, if the midwife had cared for a woman who had a particularly interesting or unusual obstetric history. The midwife would be able to focus in detail on issues of interest and make recommendations for others who may come across a similar case.

Box 7.3   Is a case study is the most appropriate tool?

- Will the case study be of relevance or interest to midwives, users of the maternity services or other health professionals?
- Do you have access to the individual concerned and all relevant documentation (e.g. case notes, pregnancy hand-held records, midwifery notes)?
- How will you protect the individual's confidentiality when presenting the case study?

Table 7.3   Example of a case study

Authors	Aim of study	Tools used
Woods (1994)	To describe a model of care to aid midwifery decision-making when caring for women in labour.	Review of birth plan.

Ways of collecting data

Questionnaires

Many midwives will be familiar with questionnaires, which are frequently used in research. They can be used to collect quantitative or qualitative data, or a combination of both. One reason for questionnaires being so commonly used is their adaptability – a researcher can design a questionnaire to suit whatever question is posed and whatever the intended population. However questionnaire design can be very time-consuming.

Attention has to be paid to ensure that questions are clear, unbiased and relevant to answer the research question (see Chapter 15).

In a study to investigate the morbidity of childbirth (MacArthur et al 1991), a postal questionnaire was sent to women between 1 and 9 years after they had given birth to ask about their experience of health problems. If a woman had one or more of the 25 health problems listed in the questionnaire, she was asked to answer more specific questions. Each time she ticked 'yes' she had to go on to answer the next question. For example:

a) Did you have this condition before the baby's birth? (YES/NO)
b) How long after having the baby did it start or come back?
c) After how long did you stop having it?
d) Did you go to the doctor? (YES/NO)
e) What treatment did you have?

Over 11 000 women returned the questionnaire. Health problems which fulfilled strict inclusion criteria (the woman had to report a new symptom which occurred within 3 months of the index delivery and lasted for over 6 weeks) were linked to each woman's obstetric case notes to look for possible causal associations with maternal, obstetric or anaesthetic characteristics.

The study showed for the first time the extent and persistence of health problems after childbirth; 47% of the women had one or more new health problems, 60% of whom reported that the symptom was still present at the time of enquiry. The study provides an excellent example of the amount of data that can be generated from a well-designed questionnaire that asks

---

Box 7.4 Is a questionnaire is the most appropriate tool?

- Are all the questions included relevant to the aim of your study?
- Have you included any questions that may cause embarrassment or anxiety?
- Are your questions clear and unbiased?
- What is the most appropriate location or method to put the questionnaire to your target population?
- Do you have financial resources available to pay for any printing and postage costs?
- How will you code and analyse the data?

Table 7.4 Examples of studies which have used questionnaires

Authors	Aim of study	Tools used
MacArthur et al (1991)	To investigate women's long-term health problems after childbirth.	Obstetric case note review.
Chamberlain et al (1993)	To obtain women's views about different approaches to pain relief during labour.	Obstetric case note review.

relevant questions. The findings resulted in subsequent studies to assess postnatal health and care (Bick and MacArthur 1995, Bick et al 1997).

Using a questionnaire has many advantages for the researcher.

- They are relatively inexpensive to produce.
- They can be an efficient use of the researcher's time in that they can be administered to a large sample of people at the same time (as in the example above).
- Respondents may provide more accurate information, as they are not facing a researcher who is asking them direct questions.

However, consideration should be given to minimize some disadvantages. For example, there may be a low response rate either because respondents do not understand questions or may not consider them relevant. These issues must be considered carefully before deciding if a questionnaire should be used.

Interviews

This tool involves direct questioning of participants either individually or as part of a group. Information can be collected using an *unstructured*, *semi-structured* or *structured* format. Interview data can be enhanced by using other tools, including questionnaires, diaries or a case note review (see Chapter 16).

An unstructured interview would be used when the researcher has no pre-specified idea of the type of information which could be collected or does not want to impose their own preconceived ideas or priorities on a research topic. For example, if the research question was to find out what factors affected pregnant women's smoking behaviour, an unstructured interview would enable respondents to describe fully their opinions or feelings on what affected their smoking behaviour. This information would be captured using a tape recorder or by writing the interviewee's comments down verbatim. 'Themes' identified from the transcribed tape or field notes would be used to describe factors that contributed to the research area of interest and possibly to develop hypotheses that could be tested using quantitative methods.

Another way to find out about women's smoking behaviour would be to conduct structured or semi-structured interviews. A structured interview would involve the researcher asking a sample of women the same set of questions (for example, 'How long have you been smoking?' 'Does anything affect the number of cigarettes you smoke in a day?' 'Have you ever tried to stop smoking?'). Questions could be asked either during face-to-face interviews or read out to women over the telephone. A semi-structured interview would involve asking the women *closed* and *open* questions – in other words there would be some questions that each

---

Box 7.5   Is interviewing is the most appropriate tool?

- Do you have sufficient time to conduct interviews?
- Do you have access to the intended study participants? If not, how will you gain access?
- Could your presence as an 'interviewer' (a health professional) influence the participant's (the consumer or a fellow health professional's) answers?
- Are you confident that you will be able to record accurately your interviews by tape or the taking of verbatim notes?
- How will you code and analyse the data?

Table 7.5   Examples of studies which have used interviews

Authors	Aim of study	Other tools used
Nolan and Hicks (1997)	To establish whether there were variations in the philosophy and approach of three groups of childbirth teachers.	None.
Creasy (1997)	To investigate women's experiences of transfer from community-based to consultant-based maternity care	None.

woman would be asked to answer specifically, but the interviewer would also ask a woman for her views about certain matters and she would be able to respond freely.

Observation

Particular research questions may not be answered fully by interviews or questionnaires that rely on the respondent to report what they think or what they do. Observation of the natural setting (such as the ward, clinic or delivery room) may provide the data required. This is a particularly useful tool if the researcher wishes to compare the information that a participant has provided in a questionnaire or during an interview with what actually happens in practice. For example an observational study would present the researcher with an excellent opportunity to observe, relatively unobtrusively, the interactions of midwives who may have reported at interview that they always seek the permission of a woman in labour before carrying out any procedure.

The researcher takes notes during the period of observation. Notes can be collected using a prepared checklist or taken down verbatim to provide the basis of a narrative account. A checklist would enable the researcher to record whether a defined list of activities they wished to observe actually took place. If a qualitative approach is used, the observer is not constrained to note only certain phenomena or types of behaviour. Field notes can be made during the period of observation, or can be written up as soon as possible afterwards (see Chapter 17).

Participant observation is used if the researcher wants to interact with the study group being observed. The researcher will have a high degree of contact and involvement with the study participants. The study undertaken by Hunt & Symonds (1995) is an excellent example of this. The aim of the study, which was conducted over a 6-month period, was to examine the practice of midwives working at two maternity units. The importance of the researcher not taking on a 'clinical' role which could have affected the situation being observed is clearly described by the authors.

If observation is the appropriate tool to answer a question about practice, specific ethical issues have to be considered. The researcher will have to decide if the women and staff should be informed that they are part of a study, as this may alter their behaviour during the period of observation. However, not informing someone that research is taking place and not obtaining their permission to observe them, is contrary to the principle of informed consent (See Chapter 4 for a discussion of ethical issues).

Box 7.6   Is observation is the most appropriate tool?

- Could your presence as an observer influence the behaviour of those being observed?
- Are you aware of your own biases or prejudices, which may influence your interpretation of what you are observing? For example, you are observing a midwife in the delivery suite who performs continuous CTG monitoring on a woman in labour. This is something you would not routinely do.
- Have you considered ethical problems, which may arise if individuals are not asked for their permission to be included in the study?
- How will observation data be coded and analysed?

Table 7.6   Examples of observation studies

Authors	Aim of study	Other tools used
Kirkham (1989)	To observe midwives and information-giving during labour.	Interviews.
Hunt & Symonds (1995)	To explore the working practices and culture of two maternity units	Interviews.

Diaries

Diaries completed by the study sample are a valuable way of obtaining detailed information. Events, symptoms or activities can be recorded to provide quantitative and/or qualitative data. As part of an observational study of the perceptions of student midwives during their initial encounters in a school of midwifery, students were asked to keep a diary to record their experiences of daily events in the clinical setting (Davies

1996). In a survey to examine postnatal care during the first 8 weeks after childbirth, women were asked to fill in a diary every fourth day until day 12 to describe any social or emotional problems they had and to record details of care received from midwives (Marchant & Garcia 1996). It is important that clear instructions are provided for the respondents so they know what is required of them (Oppenheim 1992).

Box 7.7   Is a diary is the most appropriate tool?

- If a diary is unstructured, have you considered how confidentiality can be assured when reporting results?
- Are you confident that respondents will have the time and the motivation to keep a diary record?
- How will you code and analyse data?

Table 7.7   Examples of studies which have used diaries

Authors	Aim of study	Other tools used
Marchant & Garcia (1996)	To record in detail the events of the early postnatal period.	Interviews, questionnaires. One page calendar.
Davies (1996)	Study of perceptions of student midwives during their initial encounters in a school of midwifery.	Interviews.

SUMMARY

Undertaking research can be extremely rewarding, particularly if findings lead to an improvement in care for women and their babies, or inform evidence-based midwifery knowledge and practice. As research is a recent phenomenon in midwifery, some midwives may feel anxious that they do not possess research skills. Undertaking research does mean learning new skills – it requires that thought is given to the question, that the relevant literature is reviewed and that consideration is given to the most appropriate method to answer the question. Seek the advice of others whose expertise may strengthen the study approach. Prepare to be flexible, as often, when a question is explored in detail, a different research pathway is indicated. The maternity services have undergone many changes over recent decades, which were not evidence-based. As midwives we should not allow our practice to develop without research evidence to support what we do.

Box 7.8   Questions for discussion and personal reflection

- How many areas of your practice are evidence-based?
- Think of an area of your practice that you feel requires research to evaluate its effectiveness and benefit.
  - What question would you ask?
  - What method and tools would you use to answer the question?
  - Why would this method and these tools be the most appropriate?
  - Would other professionals be able to assist you?

FURTHER READING

Bowling A *Research Methods in Health. Investigating health and health services* Milton Keynes: Open University Press; 1997
Quantitative and qualitative methods are described clearly and concisely. The book is aimed at researchers from a range of different disciplines.
Cartwright A *Health Surveys in Practice and Potential: a critical review of their scope and methods* London: King's Fund Publishing Office; 1988
This book is invaluable for anyone interested in carrying out a survey. Questions, which could be answered by surveys, are described and aspects of survey methodology discussed.
Hicks CM *Undertaking Midwifery Research. A Basic Guide to Design and Analysis* New York: Churchill Livingstone; 1996
Introduces some of the most useful methods to use in midwifery research and explains how to undertake and analyse experimental studies.
Rees C *An Introduction to Research for Midwives* Hale, Cheshire: Books for Midwives Press; 1997
This book focuses on research methods and processes, critical evaluation of research and the application of research to midwifery practice. It is clearly written and easy to follow.

REFERENCES

Abdellah FG, Levine E *Preparing Nursing Research for the 21st Century. Evaluation, Methodologies, Challenges* New York: Springer Publishing Company; 1994
Bick DE, MacArthur C 'The Extent, Severity and Effect of Health Problems After Childbirth' *British Journal of Midwifery* 1995; **3(1):** 27–31
Bick DE, MacArthur C, Winter H et al 'Redesigning Postnatal Care: physical and psychological needs' *British Journal of Midwifery* 1997; **5(10):** 621–622
Bowling A *Research Methods in Health. Investigating Health and Health Services* Milton Keynes: Open University Press; 1997
Burnard P, Morrison P *Nursing Research in Action* Second edition Houndmills: Macmillan; 1994
Cartwright A *Health Surveys in Practice and Potential: a critical review of their scope and methods* London: King's Fund Publishing Office; 1988
Chamberlain G, Wraight AM, Steer P *Pain and its Relief in Childbirth* Edinburgh: Churchill Livingstone; 1993
Creasy JM 'Women's Experience of Transfer from Community-based to Consultant-based Maternity Care' *Midwifery* 1997; **13:** 32–39
Davies RM 'Practitioners in Their Own Right: an ethnographic study of the perceptions of student midwives' in Robinson S, Thomson AM *Midwives, Research and Childbirth* Volume 4 London: Chapman and Hall; 1996
Department of Health *Changing Childbirth. Report of the Expert Maternity Group.* London: HMSO; 1993

Garcia J, Redshaw M, Fitzsimmons B, Keene J *First Class Delivery. A national survey of women's views of maternity care* Abingdon, Oxford: Audit Commission Publications; 1998

Hennekins CH, Buring JE *Epidemiology in Medicine* Boston/Toronto: Little, Brown and Company; 1987

House of Commons Select Committee *Second Report on Maternity Services* London: HMSO; 1992

Hunt S, Symonds A *The Social Meaning of Midwifery* Houndmills: Macmillan; 1995

Kirkham M 'Midwives and Information-giving During Labour' in Robinson S, Thomson A *Midwives, Research and Childbirth* Volume 1 London: Chapman and Hall; 1989

MacArthur C, Lewis M, Knox EG *Health After Childbirth* London: HMSO; 1991

Marchant S, Garcia J 'Routine Clinical Care in the Immediate Postnatal Period' in Alexander J, Levy V, Roch S *Aspects of Midwifery Practice. A Research-Based Approach* Houndmills: Macmillan; 1996

Nolan ML, Hicks CM 'Aims, Processes and Problems of Antenatal Education as Identified by Three Groups of Childbirth Teachers' *Midwifery* 1997; **13:** 179–188

Oppenheim A *Questionnaire Design, Interviewing and Attitude Measurement* Second edition London: Pinter Publishers; 1992

Rees C *An Introduction to Research for Midwives* Hale, Cheshire: Books for Midwives Press; 1997

Rogers J, Woods J, McCandlish R, Ayers S, Truesdale A, Elbourne D 'Active Versus Expectant Management of Third Stage of Labour: the Hinchingbrooke randomized controlled trial' *The Lancet* 1998; **351:** 693–699

Sleep J, Grant A, Garcia J, Elbourne D, Spencer J, Chalmers I 'West Berkshire Perineal Management Trial' *British Medical Journal* 1984; **289(8):** 587–590

Turnbull D, Holmes A, Shields N, Cheyne H, Twaddle S, Gilmour WH et al 'Randomized Controlled Trial of Efficacy of Midwife-managed Care' *Lancet* 1996; **348:** 213–218

Woods A 'Models of Care to Help Midwives in Decision-making' *British Journal of Midwifery* 1994; **2(8):** 381–386

8

Words into action: disseminating and implementing the findings of research

Soo Downe

KEY ISSUES

- Researchers working in the field of midwifery are chiefly concerned with the use of findings to inform practice
- Translation of research evidence into practice in the maternity services has been erratic. A number of changes have occurred, and are occurring, with no firm research base to support them.
- Many clinicians find published research hard to undestand. New

developments in the interpretation and presentation of evidence may improve this situation.
- Systematic reviews do not currently provide clear information as to the best method for dissemination of research into practice.
- New developments in whole systems approaches to the implementation of evidence seem to offer a promising way forward.

INTRODUCTION

As Carolyn Hicks discovered in her study published in 1993, midwives have not been slow to take up the research agenda. Of her sample, 64% had conducted research (Hicks 1993). However, only 6% of these had had their findings published outside their own institution. Despite the fact that the percentage of those undertaking formal study in her sample was almost certainly an over estimate of research activity in the population of midwives as a whole, the results reveal a clear gap between the desire to undertake research, and the capacity to get findings into the public domain. The debate is not only, however, centred on researchers. If effective care is to become a reality, it is incumbent on midwives in clinical practice to not only look for the evidence base, but also to discuss it with colleagues, decision-makers and users of the service alike.

It is generally assumed that the most effective method of spreading the word about research results is to publish them in an academic journal. However, as Helen Roberts points out: 'Publication also means "to make entirely known". "Publication", in the narrow sense is only one part of this process, and ... may sometimes not be part of it at all' (Roberts 1984).

The premise of this chapter is that researchers working in the field of midwifery are chiefly concerned with the use of findings to inform practice. This may, unusually, be the use of startling new findings to change practice overnight, or, more commonly, may be an additional piece in a jigsaw of evidence which slowly informs developments in care. In order to fulfil this end, publication may include a variety of methods. As Mary Renfrew stated in 1997:

'... researchers have a responsibility to communicate the results of their work effectively, in a language which practitioners can understand, in journals which practitioners, managers, and policy-makers read, and at conferences attended by those with an influence on clinical care' (Renfrew 1997).

This chapter addresses the issue of dissemination of research findings, and their application in practice. It seeks to establish the problems which have been identified in getting research into practice, and to offer some solutions. It suggests methods for communicating results effectively, and it presents a brief overview of new developments in the interpretation of data which are beginning to feature in the literature. Many of the examples given are from controlled studies, but the points made apply generally.

IS RESEARCH GETTING INTO PRACTICE?

There is good evidence that, despite all the emphasis on the value of research over recent years, its application in practice has been uneven. A brief examination of this phenomenon may be instructive and may help us address the issue of the optimum method of dissemination.

Case study: routine enemas in labour

In 1980 and 1981, Mona Romney published two studies relating to intra-partum practices. The first was related to pre-delivery shaving. The second, co-authored with Hannah Gordon, related to the use of enemas in labour. Both studies were published in the *British Medical Journal*. This case study focuses on the second piece of research. At the time, the use of enemas in the first stage of labour was widespread, but it had never been evaluated. Mona Romney was one of the very first midwife researchers to design and conduct a randomized, controlled trial, and, thus, to face the problems inherent in undertaking such a venture. Her paper illustrated the resistance to the study from both midwives and obstetricians, who could not believe that research would tell them anything that they did not know already about the practice. However, once the midwives perceived that women who had received an enema experienced more soiling and discomfort, they refused to continue giving the treatment to those in the intervention group. As a consequence, the study was stopped prematurely. The final report indicated that there was no real difference between the groups. The findings were taken up by the media, and by lay support groups such as

AIMS (AIMS 1981). They were also reinforced by a less widely quoted randomized controlled trial reported by Drayton and Rees in 1984.

In the same year that the Drayton and Rees study was published, Sally Garforth and Jo Garcia undertook a national survey of maternity policies in all English health districts. The study was called 'Policy and Practice in Midwifery' (Garcia et al 1987). They examined a number of aspects of maternity care, including pre-delivery shaving and the use of enemas (Garforth & Garcia 1987). The study had a 93% response rate from directors of maternity services and revealed that a policy of 'no routine bowel preparation' was only in existence in 16% of maternity units. At the other extreme, 16% had a policy of routine bowel preparation. Most units had a policy relating to specific reasons, or individual clinician's decisions. Given this fact, it is of interest that, when asked to estimate the proportion of women having bowel preparation in their units, only 35% responded 'hardly any'. This suggests that the hands-on practitioner, usually a midwife, was often making a decision in favour of an enema, despite the evidence which was then current. When asked why an enema was not used, none of the quoted responders mentioned any research. One, however, made the following comment: 'We don't give one unless it is requested. It is not routine because we have some radical midwives here' (Garcia and Garforth 1987).

This statement raises the issue of the role of opinion leaders, and this topic is returned to later in this chapter.

Since the Policy and Practice in Midwifery study, three further national studies of maternity care have been conducted. Anne Jacoby published a survey which was also undertaken in 1984. This found that 39% of all 1408 women responding to the question about whether they had an enema in labour responded that they had. Of those who had not wanted one 28% did, in fact, receive one (Jacoby 1987). The most recent reports published in England, both national reviews, do not mention the use of enemas, either in hospital protocols (Clinical Standards Advisory Group 1995) or in women's experience (Garcia et al 1998). The demise of the practice is further reinforced by the inclusion of the enema in the table relating to 'practices which may be harmful and should be discontinued' in the *Guide to Effective Care in Pregnancy and Childbirth* (Enkin et al 1995). This suggests that the subject is no longer contentious.

However, a review by the World Health Organization, published in 1996, comments on the fact that 'enemas are still widely used' (WHO 1996), and goes on to illustrate the evidence base, which remains that of the Romney and Gordon and Drayton and Rees studies. Clearly, there has been a local, but not an international impact of this work, and the key source of information is still the original articles. Enemas are noted in the WHO document as practices which are clearly harmful and should be eliminated. However, the most recent Cochrane entry on the subject is in

---

Box 8.1 Linking evidence and practice

- What do you think were the driving forces behind the reduction in the use of enemas over time in the UK?
- Why does practice seem to be more resistant to change elsewhere?
- If you were practising in an environment where routine enemas were still given, what strategies would you adopt, either as a researcher or as a clinician, to inform colleagues about the evidence in this area?

---

protocol form only (Cuervo et al 1998), and the results of any quality review on the subject will be of interest.

What does this case study tell us? That the *right study, at the right time, in the right journal, with the right level of support from both midwives and women using the service, will change practice.* However, there are plenty of practices which have *not* changed over time *despite* the evidence, and, conversely, many which have changed in response to very little information. One example of the former is the issue of communication with labouring women. Mavis Kirkham demonstrated communication deficits between midwives and women in her thesis in 1983, and she has published widely on the subject since. Some of the problems she raised at that time were still evident in the work published by Chris Henderson in 1990, and by Hunt and Symonds in 1995.

On the other hand, non-suturing of small perineal tears, even with muscle involvement, is becoming increasingly widespread in the practice of midwives, despite the only substantial evidence on the subject arising from a controlled trial relating to the non-suturing of perineal skin, and not of the muscle layer (Gordon et al 1998). This trend echoes that of the widespread introduction of continuous electronic fetal monitoring by obstetricians, in the absence of a firm evidence base. Why have some practices changed and not others? It seems that culture is more difficult to shift than clinical practice, unless that practice (such as fetal monitoring for doctors, or non-intervention at the suturing stage for midwives) is based on fundamental beliefs, such as the value of universal surveillance, or the natural tendency of the body to heal itself.

UNDERSTANDING RESEARCH

Whatever the approach adopted by the reader of research, the published data need to be understood. The next section discusses this issue.

Making results comprehensible

Even after conducting the most rigorous of research studies the researcher is always left with the problem of analysing and explaining the results.

In the case of qualitative research, this is clearly an interpretative exercise. For experimental research, interpretation may be perceived to be an easy task, since all it involves is running a few tests and producing the results. However, this is an extremely simplistic view of data interpretation.

Horton (1995) calls attention to the so-called 'spin' that researchers can put on their results in the discussion section of their papers and warns that the linguistic tricks played by authors can lead to erroneous conclusions. In response to commentary by Trisha Greenhalgh (Greenhalgh 1995) on his original article, Horton argues that a conscious attempt to untangle this rhetoric would, far from rending the subsequent text dry and boring, lead to better implemented results. Quite apart from the way the results are written up, the use of particular mathematical tests can influence the way the data are interpreted.

Box 8.2   What do results mean?

Which of the following two (fictional) studies would be most likely to influence your practice?

A) A randomized controlled study of over 6000 women in labour with their baby in the occipito-posterior position, showed that the rate of instrumental delivery was reduced from 7.8% in the control group to 6.3% in the group who were randomized into a non-time limited second stage. This was a statistically significant difference.

B) When 7825 women in labour with their baby in the occipito-posterior position were studied in a randomized controlled trial, the use of oxytocin in the active first stage of labour reduced the overall risk of an instrumental delivery by 20% compared to those randomized to the no-oxytocin group. This difference was statistically significant. (Adapted from Forrow et al 1992)

The effect of the two treatments was, in fact, identical.

Bulpitt (1987) demonstrated that manipulation of the level of confidence interval employed, from 90% to 99%, results in quite different appearances to the data. Naylor et al (1992) presented the same set of data to three groups of clinicians and experts using three different analytic strategies. They found that the willingness of the participants to act on the results varied directly with the type of tests used. As Hux and Naylor (1995) found, this also seems to be the case for users of the service. In the latter case, acceptance of a treatment varied according to the way the data were presented from 31% (using 'number needed to treat') to 88% (using relative risk reduction). This finding illustrates the need for absolute transparency when reporting on a study, whether it is an ethnographic analysis, or a placebo-controlled, double blind, randomized controlled trial.

Even carefully controlled, run, analysed and reported studies can be misunderstood. A classic example of this is the Bristol Third Stage Trial (Prendiville et al 1988). The trial was stopped prematurely when a planned interim analysis revealed an excess of bleeding in women allocated to the physiological third stage group. The authors were careful to interpret this finding in the context of the trial, to state that the results only applied in comparable populations, and to urge that the work should be replicated in a different environment where physiological management was more prevalent. However, antagonists to the routine use of syntometrine accused the researchers of utilizing bad design, without apparently reading the authors' own interpretation of their findings (Stevenson 1989). Chalmers (1983) identifies this kind of reaction as one of the 'authoritarian strategies' used to decry the results of research. He lists the strategies employed by antagonists to such enquiry, who come from both the clinical and lay perspectives. These strategies include: discussion of the ethics of withholding treatment; the need for fully informed consent; the application of the results in practice; criticisms of design; and criticisms of the intent of the investigators. Chalmers states that scientific enquiry, epitomized by, although not limited by, controlled studies, is, by its nature, antiauthoritarian, since it is predicated on the principle of uncertainty. This claim may be theoretically sound, but it is open to criticism, since there is plenty of evidence in practice that the design and conduct of research in general, and particularly of clinical trials, has been profoundly paternalistic, and biased by the personal views and attitudes of those running the studies. The interpretation of results into clinical practice is therefore problematic, both for the researcher, and for the clinician. The interpretation of results by trial participants and service users is very under-researched. One of the current debates is explored in the next section.

Understanding significance

Basic statistical testing, using so-called significance values, relies on knowing a number of facts about the data, such as the nature of its distribution. Statistical analysis is designed to minimize the risk of stating that a difference found in a particular study can be generalized to everyone, if in fact it was only a chance finding. The use and misuse of significance testing, and the consequent calculation of probability ('p') values, has exercised the minds of many statisticians and researchers. Two views appear to predominate: firstly that the p value is an all or nothing concept and should be rigidly applied. Supporters of this view usually contend that a value greater than the conventional 0.05 implies that the results are not significant and, therefore, not useful. Conversely, a value smaller than 0.05 implies that the findings are bound to be applicable to practice (Dar et al 1994). Other commentators reject this absolutist view and point out that the *size* of the difference between the treatments compared and the *confidence limits* around that effect are equally, if not more, important, in terms of judging the applicability of a treatment (Gardner & Altman 1986,

Bulpitt 1987). This more relativist view emphasizes the clinical decision-making necessary in interpretation of trial results. Salsburg (1990) makes the following point:

'There is no "correct" [approach]. Scientific reasoning consists of attempts to fit the complexities of reality into models useful for the organization of observations ... some fit for the time being until we can find one that fits better, or until the lack of fit begins to trouble us. But we must always recognize that we fit our observations to very arbitrary models, and we must be prepared to abandon a model if it leads to nonsense.' (Salsburg 1990).

Presentation of results in terms of the dimensions and range of effect are achieving central prominence in the cutting edge analyses of today, particularly in relation to meta-analyses and in the context of evidence-based medicine. This is demonstrated by journals such as *Bandolier* and *Evidence-Based Medicine*, and in the Cochrane Collaboration databases. These presentations include the use of the concept of 'numbers needed to treat' (NNT) (Laupacis et al, 1988, Chatellier et al 1996), and 'numbers needed to harm' (NNH) (Laupacis et al 1988, Dowie 1998). These are simple calculations of the *absolute* difference in benefit or harm between the experimental and control group. They indicate how many individuals would have to be treated compared to the controls for one of them to benefit positively from the treatment, or to be harmed by it. Such measures move away from the sometimes misleading use of percentages, and even:odds ratios and relative risk (Forrow et al 1992, Naylor et al 1992, Bucher et al 1994).

Will the audience understand?

The issue of how expert a reader needs to be in order to interpret data for clinical practice, as well as in understanding the other complexities of research method and design, is of importance in deciding how to present trial results. There is as yet no easy answer to this problem. Authors of quantitative studies should give as much data as possible to allow for later inclusion in a meta-analysis. Those reporting qualitative work should record participant characteristics, reason for their inclusion, and the process by which the final summaries are arrived at, including the base coding system.

The use of complex language in qualitative studies may also be off-putting for the users of research. Unfortunately, this extends even into the literature which is attempting to encourage research into practice, as the following quote illustrates:

'Scientific pluralism in nursing provides on the one hand a rich array of knowledge about human phenomena and ways of dealing with nursing problems while on the other a set of theoretical choices available for knowledge use in practice' (Kim 1993).

Box 8.3 Divining meaning
What does the above quote mean? Could there be a simpler way of putting it?

A rule of thumb could be that the majority of an article should be comprehensible on the first read to an average midwife working in the clinical area. Perhaps a scientific crystal mark should be developed for the dissemination of evidence.

DISSEMINATION

Where to publish?

This section presents some of the issues to be taken into account in choosing the most appropriate place to publish results.

Within the work place

This option is often forgotten, but it is important that findings are disseminated locally if the idea is truly to change practices. If it can't be done in the local setting, it is unlikely that it will be done in a wider scale.

Conferences

These can be local, national or international. The presentation may be accepted following submission in response to a call for papers, or it may be commissioned. Consider the audience, and the likely knowledge they have about the method you have used. Be transparent.

Journals

There are many imperatives to produce academic papers these days. The most potent is the Research Assessment Exercise, whereby universities are graded, and funded, partly on the evidence of publication in research journals. This is the extreme end of a 'publish or die' mentality which holds that dissemination should be via the written word, and ideally in a peer reviewed journal. This restriction aside, it is important to choose the journal carefully. In 1987, the American Ad Hoc Working Group for Critical Appraisal of the Medical Literature examined papers written in the late 1970s and early 1980s which stated that there were then over 2 million articles published in the biomedical literature in over 20 000 journals. The information explosion over the last decade guarantees that this figure has increased. If it is the intention that research should influence the clinical agenda, the choice of publication is essential. The balance is between an academic journal, which gives a study credibility, but which may not reach the wider clinical audience, and a more popular journal which will allow many readers to become aware of the work, but which may limit its uptake in other contexts. A combination of both would maximize coverage. Citation of the contents of the journal in a commonly used database, such as Midline or Cinahl, is also an important consideration.

Lay literature

There is an increasing awareness of the power of the so-called consumer in the utilization and dissemination of research results (PACE 1996, Longo et al 1997). As a bulletin from the King's Fund based Promoting Action for Clinical Effectiveness project (PACE) states, 'patients can encourage appropriate care and challenge non-evidence based practice' (PACE 1998).

Talking at conferences arranged by pressure and support groups, presenting findings to key workers, and collaborating on the dissemination of evidence, are all effective strategies in advancing the evidence-based agenda.

Media

Newspapers, radio and television should be used carefully. There are both risks and benefits to using the popular media, as Helen Roberts points out (Roberts, 1984). In her case, uptake by the popular media produced two different results. In one, negative reporting potentially reinforced damaging stereotypes about the women involved in her work. The other publication, in the apparently rather obscure magazine *Home and Freezer*, created a widespread interest in the study being reported from local mothers. The rewards of using the popular media can be unexpected, but valuable. However it is wise to remember that the media love a good story, and it is incumbent on researchers to ensure that any evidence they do release to the press is sound.

Electronic media

Many journal editors are beginning to realize that evidence-based practice cannot be facilitated by simply presenting the results of research. Often space is at a premium, and only the key messages and details of any study can be printed. The letters page has traditionally been the source of debate on research. The *British Journal of Obstetrics and Gynaecology*, for instance, routinely invites original authors to comment on letters submitted in response to their papers. Some journals, such as the American midwifery journal *Midwifery Today* have placed selected items on the Internet. A few journal editors have moved on from this, and are now beginning to produce electronic facilities to permit comment on articles. The *BMJ* and the *Lancet* both have interactive sites accessible via the Internet. This is one of the exciting new developments in the field of dissemination.

Evidence for effective dissemination

Over the last few years there has been a massive expansion of interest in effective methods of dissemination. A number of reviews of such methods have been produced, and some of them are summarized in Table 8.1.

These findings result from a simple search, and there may be many more such studies which were not identified. However, they illustrate the fact that the optimum approach to changing practice is still not well understood.

There is a national R&D programme, *'The evaluation of methods to promote the implementation of research findings'*, which illustrates this fact. The most recent Internet posting (dated February 1998) reveals that the programme has generated four complete studies to date, and 30 which are on-going. A number of these are of interest to midwives, most notably the work by Jenny Hewison, exploring the uptake of effective practices in maternity units.

Other studies will assess the cultural barriers to change. An example is the work led by John Newton in Oxford who is examining social networks and the use of research in clinical practice. The project promises to test a theory on dissemination which is currently in favour, namely the theory of *diffusion*. This is based on the well-known premise that the population can be divided into innovators, early adopters, and those who lag behind. The theory also recognizes stages in the process such as knowledge, persuasion, decision, implementation, and confirmation (Rogers 1995).

Rogers notes that an innovation is likely to be accepted if it shows a relative advantage over another practice, fits with previous experience and beliefs, is easy to understand, if the individual can experiment with it, and if the practice is very visible to others. Such an innovation, he suggests, will be easily adopted. The issue of the appropriate method of publication to choose becomes important in this context, since it has been evident since at least the early 1950s that, at least at the initial time of communication, information is more easily accepted from a trustworthy source (Hovland and Weiss 1951/2).

The diffusion theory was further explored by McKinlay in 1981 who called for an examination of the pre-diffusion phase. He commented on the nature of medical innovations, stating that the innovator is usually inspired by an enthusiastic report, which then progresses into medical practice, either through public acclaim, or professional support, or both. It then becomes difficult to evaluate, and any negative results are dismissed as

Table 8.1 Reviews of methods of dissemination of research findings

Source	Method	Subject	Conclusion	Reference
Effective Health Care bulletin	systematic review	Implementing clinical practice guidelines.	Guidelines can change practice. They need to be developed taking into account local circumstances, disseminated 'by an active educational intervention', and backed up with practice specific reminders.	*Effective Health Care Bulletin* (1994) no 8
Evidence-Based Medicine	meta-analysis	Computerized reminders in preventative services.	Computerized reminders worked in most of the areas surveyed.	Shea, DuMouchel & Bahamonde (1997)
Cochrane Library (Effective practice and organization of care group)	systematic review	Printed educational materials: effect on physician behaviours and patient outcomes.	Printed educational material on its own had no obvious benefit. With other strategies, the evidence was uncertain.	Freemantle et al (1998)
Cochrane Library (Effective practice and organization of care group)	systematic review and meta-analysis	Audit and feedback to improve professional practice and health care outcomes (part I).	Audit with feedback can sometimes have a moderate, though potentially worthwhile effect. It should be used with other techniques.	Thomson et al (1998a)
Cochrane Library (Effective practice and organization of care group)	systematic review and meta-analysis	Effect of the method of audit and feedback.	There is little evidence on mode, the content, source, timing, and format. Some evidence indicates that reminders may be useful.	Thomson et al (1998b)
Cochrane Library (Effective practice and organization of care group)	systematic review and meta-analysis	Outreach visits to improve professional practice and health care outcomes.	Educational outreach visits combined with other interventions seem to reduce inappropriate prescribing. The effects are moderate. The timing of the intervention, and the sustainability of the impact, are not clear.	Thomson et al (1998c)
Cochrane Library (Effective practice and organization of care group)	systematic review and meta-analysis	The effect of local opinion leaders.	The area is difficult and unclear. There appear to be mixed effects on practice, but more work is needed to clarify if opinion leaders can be identified, and how they can be influential.	Thomson et al (1998d)
Cochrane Library (Effective practice and organization of care group)	systematic review and meta-analysis	Impact of mass media on health services utilization.	the nature of the research in the area is poor, but such results as there are offer promise that this could be one of the useful tools.	Grilli et al (1998)

being due to a badly designed study. Over time, however, enthusiasm wanes as the technique is seen to be less than robust. Eventually (but not usually before there is an equally promising alternative), the practice falls from grace and is phased out. Ian Graham illustrated precisely this process in an in-depth exploration of the rise and fall of the use of episiotomy (Graham 1997). Some elements of the resistance phase can be seen in the negative criticism levelled by some clinicians against the studies of active versus physiological third stage management as outlined earlier. Given this tendency, it is vital that anyone reporting research is careful about the extent to which the claims made can be justified, and is transparent about the processes undertaken, whatever the method employed in the work. Practitioners reading reports should be aware of their prior biases and constructively critical of their own evaluation, before discussing its implementation into clinical practice with colleagues and managers.

RESEARCH INTO PRACTICE: CURRENT AND FUTURE APPROACHES

Hodnett and colleagues set up a carefully designed implementation RCT study within the maternity services in Canada (Hodnett et al 1996). They planned to assess the effects of opinion leaders (termed 'educational influentials') in a technique termed a 'marketing strategy'. This was based on a cohort approach, and used case and control sites. The intention was to use evidence from RCTs in an effort to change practice. At the end of the study, there were no discernible differences between the staff at the case and control sites in terms of their general knowledge base and practice. The authors attribute this to a number of reasons, including the possibility that the organizational structure and culture did not allow for change.

In an attempt to adopt an integrated approach to dissemination, the Ontario Health Care Evaluation Network (OHCEN) was set up to facilitate the transfer of research results using a policy of active dissemination (Sibbald & Kossuth 1998). The project recognized some key barriers to research. These were that decision-makers did not have access to, see the need for, understand, believe, or have the capacity to act upon research results. Similar barriers were identified amongst midwives in the studies undertaken by Hicks (1995) and Meah et al (1996). The OHCEN also took into account the fact that researchers did not usually include dissemination in their original research plan, did not choose topics which interested decision-makers, did not communicate with decision-makers, and were reluctant to undertake contract rather than peer-reviewed work. They set up an electronic forum, an annual conference, and an informatics project via the Internet. These systems were designed to bring together producers and consumers of research. The project also involved the local development of a project which set out to produce collaborative guidelines.

The whole enterprise addresses the increasing recognition of the need to adopt a 'whole systems' view, and to use multi-media solutions for dissemination. Results are not yet available, but the design may prove to be an innovative approach to the future of effective clinical practice.

CONCLUSION

MacIntyre and Porter (1989) point out that many of the problems arising in getting evidence into practice may be based in conflicting goals, with some of the objectives of providers, managers and users of care being mutually incompatible. The authors warn against over-enthusiastic adoption of innovations, or inappropriate interpretation of research findings. They state that:

'Effective maternity care takes place in a social context, and is not simply the delivery of well-validated forms of care with technical excellence. There is also a need to take into account social relationships, social and psychological processes, and concepts such as hierarchy, autonomy, status, power, vested interests, and charisma.' (MacIntyre and Porter 1989)

This chapter has explored a number of aspects of dissemination. The way the data are presented, and the credibility and accessibility of the arena in which they are published have been examined. Current developments in the communication of evidence, and possible future techniques and technologies have been presented. Some of the methods for ensuring that good quality evidence is produced, and appropriately disseminated and interpreted, may be summarized as follows:

- Research undertaken should be relevant to practice.
- Results should be disseminated transparently.
- The methods of dissemination should be chosen to maximize cover and credibility.
- Organizations should support inquisitive practitioners.
- Clinicians should take the need to disseminate and discuss evidence with colleagues seriously.

In interpreting and disseminating research evidence, it is incumbent on both researchers and clinicians to consider the effects of their chosen approach on their own practice, that of their colleagues, and, most importantly, on the women and families they care for.

FURTHER READING

Cochrane Collaboration on Effective Professional Practice Group. Available from: the Cochrane Library, Update Software, PO Box 696, Oxford OX2 7YX, England. On line from: http://www.cochrane.co.uk
This sub-group of the Cochrane Collaboration is concerned with reviews of controlled studies which explore methods of getting research into practice.

Dowie J 'Evidence-based', 'cost-effective' and 'preference-driven' medicine: decision analysis based medical decision making is the pre-requisite' *Journal of Health Service Research Policy* 1996; **1(2):** 104–113
A review of various approaches to effective clinical practice.

Lilford RJ, Pauker SG, Braunholtz DA, Chard J 'Decision analysis and the implementation of research findings'. *British Medical Journal* 1998; **317:** 405–9
Offers a method of uniting evidence based practice with the preferences of those using the service.

Dunning M, Abi-Aad G, Gilbert D, Hutton H, Brown B *Experience evidence and everyday practice: creating systems for delivering effective health care.* King's Fund, London; 1999
A summary of the outputs of the promoting action on clinical effectiveness (PACE) project. It offers general lessons from the programme as a whole, and specific case studies.

Gustafson DH, McTavish FM, Boberg E et al 'Empowering patients using computer based health support systems' *Quality in Health Care* 1999; **8(1):** 49–56
Provides a summary of an on-line evidence based information system for women with breast cancer: a thorough and user-friendly innovation which may be usefully generalised not only to other conditions for service users, but also to health professionals.

Oakley A 'Who's afraid of the randomized controlled trial? Some dilemmas of the scientific method and 'good' research practice' *Women & Health* 1989; **15(4):** 25–59
Offers a thoughtful and detailed analysis of the nature of evidence and of its value to clinical practice.

Sackett DL, Haynes RB, Guyatt GH, Tugwell P *Clinical epidemiology: a basic science for clinical medicine,* Second edition. Little, Brown, London; 1991
One of the classic texts on evidence-based medicine

Spiegelhalter DJ, Myles JP, Jones DR, Abrams KR 'An introduction to bayesian methods in health technology assessment' *British Medical Journal* 1999; **319:** 508–512
A review of the rather controversial bayesian approach to evidence. The article is rather dense, but it offers one of the few relatively accessible explorations of this topic.

'Trip' database:
http://www.gwent.nhs.gov.uk/trip/
A useful on-line gateway into a wide range of resources for evidence-based practice.

REFERENCES

Ad Hoc Working Group for Critical Appraisal of Medical Literature 'A Proposal for a More Informative Abstracting of Clinical Articles *Ann Intern Med* 1987; **106:** 598–604
AIMS *Association for Improvements in the Maternity Services Quarterly Newsletter* 1981; Autumn: 16
Bucher HC, Wienbacher M, Gyr K 'Influence of Method of Reporting Study Results on Decisions of Physicians to Prescribe Drugs to Lower Cholesterol Concentrations *BMJ* 1994; **309:** 761–764
Bulpitt CJ 'Confidence intervals' *Lancet* 1987; **1:** 494–497
Chalmers I 'Scientific Enquiry and Authoritarianism in Perinatal Care and Education' *Birth* 1983; **10(3):** 151–165
Chatellier G, Zapletal E, Lemaitre D, Menard J, Degoulet P 'The Number Needed to Treat: a clinically useful normogram in its proper context' *BMJ* 1996; **312:** 426–429
Clinical Standards Advisory Group *Women In Normal Labour* Report of a CSAG Committee on Women in Normal Labour; 1995
Cuervo LG, Rodriguez MN, Delgado MB 'Enema vs no Enema During Labor' in Neilson JP, Crowther CA, Hodnett ED, Hofmeyr GJ *Pregnancy and Childbirth Module of The Cochrane Database of Systematic Reviews* The Cochrane Collaboration; Issue 1. Oxford: Update Software; 1998
Dar R, Serlin RC, Omer H 'Misuse of Statistical Tests in Three Decades of Psychotherapy Research' *J Consult Clin Psychol* 1994; **62(1):** 75–82
Dowie J 'The "number needed to treat" and the "adjusted NNT" in health care decision-making' *J Health Serv Res Policy* 1998; **3(1):** 44–49

Drayton S, Rees C 'They know what they're doing' Nursing Mirror (Midwifery Forum) 1984; **159**: 4–8

Effective Healthcare Bulletin Implementing Clinical Practice Guidelines. Bulletin no 8. Nuffield Institute for Health/University of Leeds Centre for Health Economics/NHS Centre for Reviews and Dissemination University of York; 1994

Enkin M, Keirse MJNC, Renfrew M, Neilson J A Guide to Effective Care in Pregnancy and Childbirth Oxford: Oxford University Press; 1995

Forrow L, Taylor WC, Arnold RM 'Absolutely Relative: how research results are summarized can affect treatment decisions' Am J Med 1992; **92**: 121–124

Freemantle N, Harvey EL, Grimshaw JM, Grilli R, Bero LA 'Printed Educational Materials to Improve the Behaviour of Health Care Professionals and Patient Outcomes' in Bero L, Grilli R, Grimshaw J, Oxman A Collaboration on Effective Professional Practice Module of the Cochrane Database of Systematic Reviews The Cochrane Collaboration Issue 1 Oxford: Update Software; 1998

Garcia J, Garforth S, Ayers S 'The Policy and Practice in Midwifery Study: introduction and methods' Midwifery 1987; **3**: 2–9

Garcia J, Redshaw M, Fitsimons B, Kenne J First Class Delivery: A national survey of women's views of maternity care Audit Commission: National Perinatal Epidemiology Unit; 1998

Gardner MJ, Altman DG 'Confidence Intervals Rather Than P Values: estimation rather than hypothesis testing' BMJ 1986; **292**: 746–750

Garforth S, Garcia J 'Admitting – a weakness or a strength? Routine admission of a woman in labour' Midwifery 1987; **3(1)**: 10–24

Gordon B, Mackrodt C, Fern E, Truesdale A, Ayers S, Grant A 'The Ipswich Childbirth Study: A randomised evaluation of two stage postpartum perineal repair leaving the skin unsutured' Br J Obstet Gynaecol 1998; **105**: 435–440

Graham ID Episiotomy; challenging obstetric interventions Abingdon: Blackwell Science; 1997

Greenhalgh T 'Commentary: Scientific heads are not turned by rhetoric' BMJ 1995; **310**: 987–988

Grilli R, Freemantle N, Minozzi S, Domenighetti G, Finer D 'Impact of Mass Media Campaigns on Health Services Utilization and Health Care Outcomes' in Bero L, Grilli R, Grimshaw J, Oxman A Collaboration on Effective Professional Practice Module of the Cochrane Database of Systematic Reviews The Cochrane Collaboration: Issue 1; 1998

Henderson C 'Artificial Rupture of the Membranes' in Alexander J, Levy V, Roche S Midwifery Practice vol 2 Oxford: Macmillan Education Ltd; 1990

Hicks C 'A Factor Analytic Study of Midwives' Attitudes to Research' Midwifery 1995; **11**: 11–17

Hicks C 'A Survey of Midwives' Attitudes to, and Involvement in, Research: the first stage in identifying needs for a staff development programme' Midwifery 1993; **9**: 51–62

Hodnett E, Kaufman K, O'Brien-Pallas L, Chipman M, Watson-MacDonnell J, Hunsburger W 'A Strategy to Promote Research-based Nursing Care: effects on childbirth outcomes' Research in Nursing and Health 1996; **19**: 13–20

Horton R 'The Rhetoric of Research' BMJ 1995; **310**: 985–987

Hovland CI, Weiss W 'The Influence of Source Credibility on Communication Effectiveness' Public Opinion Quarterly Winter: 1951–1952

Hunt S, Symonds A The social meaning of midwifery London: Macmillan; 1995

Huy JF, Naylor CD 'Communicating the Benefits of Chronic Preventive Therapy: does the format of efficacy data determine patients' acceptance of treatment?' Medical Decision Making 1995; **15**: 152–157

Jacoby A 'Women's Preferences for Satisfaction with Current Procedures in Childbirth – findings from a national study' Midwifery 1987; **3**: 117–124

Kim HS 'Putting theory into practice: problems and prospects' Journal of Advanced Nursing 1993; **18**: 1632–1639

Kirkham M Basic supportive care in labour; interaction with and around labouring women Unpublished PhD thesis, Manchester University, Faculty of Medicine; 1987

Laupacis A, Sackett DL, Roberts RS 'An Assessment of Clinically Useful Measures of the Consequences of Treatment' The New England Journal of Medicine 1988; **318(26)**: 1728–1733

Longo DR, Land G, Schramm W, Fraas J, Hoskins B, Howell V 'Consumer Reports in Health Care: do they make a difference in patient care?' JAMA 1997; **278(19)**: 1579–1584

Macintyre S, Porter M 'Prospects and Problems in Promoting Effective Care at the Local Level' in Chalmers I, Enkin M, Keirse MJNC *Effective Care in Pregnancy and Childbirth* Oxford: Oxford University Press; 1989

McKinlay JB 'From "Promising Report" to "Standard Procedure": Seven Stages in the Career of a Medical Innovation' *Millbank Memorial Fund Quarterly/Health and Society* 1981; **59:** 3

Meah S, Luker K, Cullum N 'An Exploration of Midwives' Attitudes to Research and Perceived Barriers to Research Utilisation' *Midwifery* 1996; **12:** 73–84

Naylor CD, Chen E, Strauss B 'Measured Enthusiasm; does the method of reporting trial results alter perceptions of therapeutic effectiveness?' *Annals of Int Med* 1992; **117:** 916–921

PACE *Involving Patients* King's Fund PACE Bulletin, Special Issue, King's Fund Development Centre; Sept 1996

PACE *How to Involve Patients in Work on Clinical Effectiveness* King's Fund PACE Bulletin, King's Fund Development Centre; June 1998

Prendiville WJ, Harding JE, Elbourne DR, Stirrat, GM 'The Bristol Third Stage Trial: active versus physiological management of the third stage of labour' *BMJ* 1988; **297:** 1295–1300

Renfrew MJ 'Influencing the Development of Evidence-based Practice' *British Journal of Midwifery* 1997; **5(3):** 131–134

Renfrew MJ 'The Development of Evidence-based Practice' *British Journal of Midwifery* 1997; **5(2):** 100–104

Roberts H 'Putting the Show in the Road: the dissemination of research findings' in Bell, Roberts *Social Researching*; 1984

Rogers EM 'Lessons for guidelines from the diffusion of innovations' *Journal of Quality Improvement* 1995; **21(7):** 24–28

Romney ML, Gordon H 'Is Your Enema Really Necessary?' *British Medical Journal* 1981; **282:** 1269–1271

Salsburg D 'Hypothesis versus significance testing for controlled clinical trials: a dialogue' *Statistics in Medicine* 1990; **9(3):** 201–211

Shea S, DuMouchel W, Bahamonde L 'Review: Computerized reminders increase the rate of use of most preventative services' *Evidence-Based Medicine* 1997; **2(3):** May/ June

Sibbald WJ, Kossuth JD 'The Ontario Healthcare Evaluation Network (OHCEN) and the Critical Care Research Network as Vehicles for Research Transfer' *Medical Decision Making* 1998; **18:** 1

Stevenson J 'The Bristol Third Stage Trial: a critical review' *Association of Radical Midwives Magazine* 1989; **41:** 11–12

Thomson MA, Oxman AD, Davis DA, Haynes RB, Freemantle N, Harvey EL 'Audit and Feedback to Improve Health Professional Practice and Healthcare Outcomes (Part I)' in Bero L, Grilli R, Grimshaw J, Oxman A *Collaboration on Effective Professional Practice Module of The Cochrane Database of Systematic Reviews* The Cochrane Collection; Issue 1; Update Software; 1998a

Thomson MA, Oxman AD, Davis DA, Haynes RB, Freemantle N, Harvey EL 'Audit and Feedback to Improve Health Professional Practice and Healthcare Outcomes (Part II)' in Bero L, Grilli R, Grimshaw J, Oxman A *Collaboration on Effective Professional Practice Module of The Cochrane Database of Systematic Reviews* The Cochrane Collection; Issue 1; Update Software; 1998b

Thomson MA, Oxman AD, Davis DA, Haynes RB, Freemantle N, Harvey EL 'Outreach Visits to Improve Health Professional Practice and Health Care Outcomes' in Bero L, Grilli R, Grimshaw J, Oxman A *Collaboration on Effective Professional Practice Module of The Cochrane Database of Systematic Reviews* The Cochrane Collection; Issue 1; Update Software; 1998c

Thomson MA, Oxman AD, Davis DA, Haynes RB, Freemantle N, Harvey EL 'Local Opinion Leaders to Improve Health Professional Practice and Health Care Outcomes' in Bero L, Grilli R, Grimshaw J, Oxman A *Collaboration on Effective Professional Practice Module of The Cochrane Database of Systematic Reviews* The Cochrane Collection; Issue 1; Update Software; 1998d

World Health Organisation *Care in Normal Birth: a practical guide. Report of a Technical Working Group* World Health Organisation; 1996

9

Developing standards for practice

Julie Wray and Angie Benbow

KEY ISSUES

- Multi-professional approaches to quality and collaborative team work within the framework of clinical governance.
- The process of standard formation and clinical audit.

- Examples of auditable standards in maternity care.
- Involving women in standard development and quality issues.

INTRODUCTION

With the impact of the *Changing Childbirth* report, a national drive to create a more efficient and effective consumer-led maternity service is in process (Department of Health 1993a). This approach is further supported by the Government's determination that all patients should receive a first class service. The service is required to become more woman-centred, provide attention appropriate to women's needs, and to be accessible and effective. This will be achieved through clinical governance with an emphasis on quality and equity at the heart of health care (Department of Health 1998a). This new style of maternity service enables midwives to reassert their position as practitioners, freeing them to manage normal pregnancy and childbirth in partnership with women. But what underpins their practice; what evidence exists? Do they audit their practice and evaluate what is best? Are they doing it right?

Midwives must not only audit and evaluate their own sphere of practice but also must participate in the audit and evaluation of other professionals' practice whenever it relates to maternity care. Communication with other health professionals is an integral part of this process and has implications for the effective use of resources, facilitating seamless care. This provides an enormous challenge for midwives who may have previously under-valued the role of clinical audit and standard development in maternity care and may not have developed the skills to evaluate it. In this chapter we build on previous themes by highlighting how research can be implemented into clinical practice by means of the clinical audit process. Our purpose is to assist midwives in identifying clinical and organizational procedures in maternity practice where sound clinical audit could improve the provision of care. This chapter is intended to be a guide, providing a framework for the audit process, the development of standards and the continuum of the audit spiral in maternity care. The philosophy is that audit should be collaborative, involving a multi-professional team and incorporating intersectoral approaches, that is integrating primary and secondary care.

QUALITY HEALTH CARE

Quality has resumed its rightful place within the NHS, with clinical governance as the new quality framework. With clinical governance NHS organizations are now accountable for continuously improving the quality of their services and safeguarding high standards of care (Department of Health 1998a). However, developing and implementing quality health care remains surprisingly complex and challenging. This process is further complicated when considering the multi-professional contributions and intersectoral approaches to care. Different sub-groups of the health care population, professionals and consumers, have different perspectives and priorities and raise different issues, all of which should theoretically add depth and strength to quality initiatives. However, developing quality initiatives, in particular clinical audit and standard development, which reflect this approach to health care can be an intricate and time consuming venture (Wray & Maresh 1997). Nevertheless, clinical audit is an area where successful implementation is likely to have significant health gains and is high on the list of priorities in the UK health service agenda of quality assurance. The recently published Government White Paper for England entitled *The New NHS* emphasizes the concept of quality assurance and clearly states '... it must be the quality of the patient experience as well as the clinical result and that quality should be measured in terms of prompt access, good relationships and efficient administration' (Department of Health 1997).

Quality within maternity care concerns practitioners taking responsibility for 'doing the right things, at the right time for the right people, and doing them right first time' (Department of Health 1997). Within a quality assurance programme, the role of clinical audit can generate useful questions about practice and clinical activity. Maternity care has the potential to be an excellent example of practitioners working closely together, creating opportunities for collaborative quality audit initiatives – but, in reality is it? It may be argued that midwives have been immersed in a role of data collection only and may have a fragmented view of clinical audit and standard setting (Wray & Maresh 1997).

AUDIT IN MATERNITY CARE

Audit in health care has been encouraged since the 1989 NHS White Paper

(Department of Health 1989) which gave audit particular impetus and promoted it as a valuable tool for improving the quality of professional care and, ultimately, patient choice (Department of Health 1989). Clinical audit in the maternity services has existed for many years, in formats such as the Confidential Enquiry into Maternal Deaths (CEMD), the National Birthday Trust surveys and, more recently, the Confidential Enquiry into Stillbirths and Deaths in Infancy (CESDI). All these reports encompass the philosophy of multi-professional approaches to the audit process. Clearly, clinical practice should be based on sound evidence and subject to regular clinical audit (Department of Health 1993b).

Medical versus clinical audit

The 1989 White Paper introduced the requirement for systematic audit of clinical practice, initially for doctors (medical audit), but later extending it to all health care professionals (clinical audit). Up until 1994, medical audit and clinical audit were seen as separate activities. Not only were these financed separately, but importantly, there was an intellectual separation. The concept of an overarching 'clinical' as opposed to 'medical' audit has been widely welcomed. Although in theory it means that all health professionals are equal when it comes to choosing the topics for audit, in reality many such topics are chosen by the medically qualified leaders of the service (Hopkins 1996). Midwives must ask themselves, have we reached the stage of professional equity in clinical audit of maternity care and are we ready? As Julia Allison stated:

'... as midwives we think we work hard, we think we give a valuable service with good outcomes, we think that we provide an economical service; but thinking is very far from knowing, when we are asked to produce statistical evidence of our achievements, we struggle to do so, because audit which is discretely related to midwives' work is not routinely undertaken.'

(Allison 1991 in Campbell & Macfarlane 1994)

Across the UK there are enormous variations in midwives' roles within audit activity. These range from audit leadership to data collection to minimal activity. The development of the role of midwives in a number of NHS Trusts has enabled midwives to participate actively in audit activities and standard setting over the past 3 years. Data available

---

Box 9.1

The Royal College of Obstetricians and Gynaecologists Clinical Audit Unit has up-to-date data on numbers and types of maternity units throughout the UK:

- 273 maternity units where births take place, of which 259 are consultant units.
- There are 114 named audit midwives who are responsible for facilitating clinical audit and related quality initiatives.

illustrates midwives' involvement across a number of maternity units across the UK (Box 9.1).

WHAT IS CLINICAL AUDIT?

Before discussing precisely how maternity care can be audited, it is necessary to clarify what clinical audit is, and is not. Clinical audit is not research. Research is finding out what is the right thing to do. Clinical audit is about finding out if the right thing is being done (Maresh 1994). However clinical audit and research share similar philosophies and methods of data collection, evidence gathering, standard setting and hypothesis testing.

'Clinical audit is a method by which we can evaluate in a systematic way the process and the outcome of the care provided. In clinical practice it is simply a structured way of looking at what we are doing, how we are doing it and the outcome of what we have done.'

(Dunn & McIlwaine 1996)

Clinical audit is a method by which all those involved in the provision and implementation of health care, including women (consumers), can evaluate, or measure, what is being provided, the processes involved in providing it and the resulting outcomes. This can be undertaken at several levels, from the individual practitioner (midwife) reviewing their own practice to multi-centred international studies. Nevertheless, wherever and however it is undertaken clinical audit is simply a formalized, structured way of looking at what we are doing, how we are doing it, and what the outcomes are, both physically and psychologically, of what we have done.

SOME KEY QUESTIONS WE NEED TO ASK ABOUT OUR PRACTICE

- What is it that we are doing?
- What is the quality of the available evidence to support this?
- Have we reached an agreement on the care we provide, or wish to provide?
- Have we set an evidence-based standard of care that we all agree on?
- How are we doing it and what methods are we using to achieve this?
- What is the evidence to support or refute these methods?
- Do we have the necessary skills, education and training to carry out these processes and are the will and the resources available to achieve these?
- What is the outcome, are we achieving the expected outcome and are the recipients and providers satisfied?

The process of clinical audit and the development of standards can help to answer these questions.

Definitions of clinical audit

There are several definitions of clinical audit and the examples in Box 9.2 highlight firstly the process of clinical audit in its broadest sense, followed by a generic, practitioner-based definition and finally a definition specific to maternity care. They all have the same philosophy in that it is the quality of care given that is important.

Box 9.2 Definitions of clinical audit

1. A broad definition of the process of clinical audit is that of a 'multi-professional, patient focused audit, leading to cost effective, high quality care delivery in clinical teams' (Batstone & Edwards 1994).
2. A more generic and often quoted definition is that 'Clinical Audit is the systematic, critical analysis of the quality of care including the procedures used for diagnosis and treatment (including prevention), the use of resources and the resulting outcome and quality of life for the patient' (Maresh 1994).
3. A definition specific to maternity care is 'Perinatal audit may be defined as: the systematic, critical analysis of the quality of perinatal care, including the procedures used for diagnosis and treatment, the use of resources and the resultant outcome and quality of life for women and their babies' (Dunn & McIlwaine 1996).

How is audit undertaken?

The process of undertaking clinical audit is important. Clinical audit that is poorly designed and implemented is at best unsettling, or even threatening, to the personnel responsible for the care being audited. At worst, services and practices could be changed on the basis of erroneous information. As clinical audit is a systematic, critical analysis of the quality of care given it requires a systematic, critical approach. There are a number of stages in undertaking clinical audit:

- Choosing a suitable topic for audit.
- Observing practice.
- Setting standards.
- Practical issues of design and implementation.
- Feedback and implementing change.

For clarity, each of the stages are addressed separately.

The stages outlined above are not mutually exclusive and they interrelate throughout the process. A diagrammatic representation is often used to show the audit process as a circle. However, it is preferable to think of this process as a *spiral* not a circle (see Figure 9.1). The spiral indicates an upward trend with improvements being made along the way and it also emphasizes the continuation of this process.

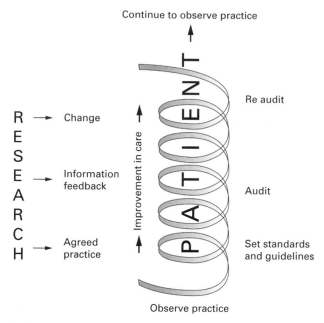

Figure 9.1 Audit spiral

Choosing a topic for audit. A topic for audit can originate from several sources. These may include the following:

• The Health Authority or the Primary Care Groups who purchase services and who may be interested in uptake of screening programmes.
• A national programme such as the drive to organize antenatal care to maximize continuity of care (Department of Health 1993b).
• The introduction of national guidelines, for example universal antenatal screening for Hepatitis B (Department of Health 1998b).
• Local initiatives, perhaps in a bid to evaluate the service offered and improve or sustain practice as appropriate.
• Following adverse events such as an increase in the rates of massive haemorrhage in the postnatal period or an increase in severe perineal trauma.
• Following media attention to a particular area of concern to women and their families, for example caesarean births, or the use of vitamin K for all newborn babies.

Box 9.3 Reflective practice

From your own clinical practice think of an aspect of care which could be audited. Why did you choose this particular topic?

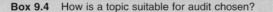

Box 9.4   How is a topic suitable for audit chosen?

When selecting topics for audit the following criteria must be met:

1. The topic must be significant either because it leads to a serious outcome, it occurs frequently, or because there is a variation in the management of care.
2. The topic must be clearly defined and the definition must be agreed by all those taking part in the audit.
3. It must be feasible to undertake the audit.
4. There must be potential to make changes as a result of audit.

(Adapted from Dunn & McIlwaine 1996)

The first stage of the audit spiral is to assess whether the topic chosen fulfils the criteria for selecting topics for audit. These criteria have been developed by the European Association of Perinatal Medicine (Dunn & McIlwaine 1996) as presented in Box 9.4.

To relate the first point to situations in midwifery:

- *It leads to a serious outcome* – for example, severe pregnancy induced hypertension.
- *It occurs frequently* – such as women reporting reduced fetal movements.
- *There is variation in the management of care between units and between practitioners* – for example the management of low risk and high risk pregnancy; are we all working to the same criteria or not?

Box 9.5   Reflective practice

Think of an audit recently undertaken in your area of practice. Why do you think this particular topic was chosen? Did it fit the above criteria? In what way?

As mentioned in Box 9.4, the topic must be defined clearly and the definition agreed on by all those taking part. This is particularly important if 'like with like' comparisons are to be made. For example, with the term 'born before arrival' (BBA); does everyone agree on the definition of what a BBA is? Does it mean 'born before arrival of the midwife or medical assistance' or 'born before arrival at booked place of birth'? There is a fundamental difference between the two. They have different meanings and implications, therefore highlighting a need for an agreed working definition.

The feasibility of undertaking the audit is an important consideration. Issues such as the availability of resources, particularly in relation to personnel availability need to be addressed. Questions that arise are:

- How easy is it to collect the required data?

- Who will design and manage the audit?
- Who will collect, enter and interpret the data?
- Who will produce and organize the feedback of a report?
- Who will be responsible for the implementation of any changes required?

Whilst an audit requires financial support, it just as importantly requires commitment from all the personnel involved.

There must be the potential to make changes as a result of the audit. If it is unlikely that changes can be made, then the amount of effort that is involved in undertaking a good quality audit will not be rewarded and may even jeopardize future audit initiatives. For instance, are resources likely to be available for feedback and implementation of any recommendations? These stages inter-relate and the issue of feedback and implementation must be discussed in the planning stages. This topic is explored further in 'Creating a culture for change' later in the chapter (page 167). However, if it is clear that an area of care would be likely to benefit from an audit, then these problems must be overcome as the results of a good quality audit can sway the staunchest challenger to alter their practice. It can also work as an excellent tool when negotiating funding.

Observing practice. Having chosen a topic which is suitable for audit, it is important to assess what happens in current practice. Who does what, to whom and when? What is the mechanism by which all this occurs? If we take the example of antenatal screening for Down's syndrome, questions that should be asked are:

- What type of screening is offered?
- Is it serum screening – double, triple, quadruple?
- Is it ultrasound – nuchal fold thickness?
- Does everyone involved know and feel confident in explaining the specificity and sensitivity of these tests?
- Are all women offered these tests or is there a criterion of risk such as age and history?
- Can women opt in or opt out of the system?
- Who gives the information to the women involved?
- Are these information givers trained and skilled to do so?
- Can they all explain risk adequately?
- What of the practical issues, such as who takes the blood samples?
- Where are they sent to?
- How long does it take to receive the results?
- What happens to the results?
- Are all women informed or only those at increased risk?
- What is considered to be high risk and what are the cut off points?
- How are the women informed of the results and what steps are in place for follow up diagnosis and counselling?

This monitoring of practice is the basis from which standards for care can be developed.

Setting standards. The foundations of high quality care are agreed standards of good clinical practice based on research evidence wherever possible.

Definition. Standards can be defined as the 'optimum level of care against which performance or adherence is compared' (Gallant & McLane 1979). In clinical practice these standards are derived from accepted evidence of the best way of delivering health care, having agreed levels of excellence.

Within the health care setting there exist organizational standards and clinical standards. Organizational standards state what facilities should be in place in order to provide a quality service and clinical standards state what procedures should be undertaken. Returning to the example of screening for Down's syndrome, examples of organizational and clinical standards are as follows:

Organizational standards:

- Written standards for all screening tests must be available (RCOG 1995a).
- All staff should be familiar with the contents of these standards and they must be readily available in antenatal clinics and GP surgeries.
- Women and their partners must be given verbal information supported by suitable written, audio-visual or audiotape information if required (Benbow et al 1997).

Clinical standards:

- The importance of an accurate gestational age e.g. obtained by ultrasound scan early in pregnancy, in calculating the level of risk (RCOG 1995b).
- All women who are offered screening for Down's syndrome will be informed of the advantages and disadvantages of the tests (Benbow et al 1997).

These standards must be dynamic and responsive to new knowledge and evidence, existing as benchmarks for the quality of service to be provided. Through clinical audit, practice can be evaluated to identify whether these standards need to be improved or redeveloped (Buckley 1997).

How to set standards. When setting standards, it is necessary to agree the level of care to be achieved. The standard should be determined by exploring the literature for current evidence. If this evidence is not available or is of ambiguous quality, then a consensus of best practice must be made. For example, in the management of threatened miscarriage, there are presently no published national guidelines in the UK to act as a framework by which standards of management can be measured (Wray & Maresh

1997). But within the framework of maternity care, a consensus of best practice will exist, even though these may differ throughout the UK. A consumer support group, the 'Miscarriage Association' have produced guidelines for good practice that are recommended for professionals and women (Moulder 1991). This highlights the benefit of a thorough investigation of the topic you are setting standards for, and the advantage of involving outside agencies that represent the users of the service. Standards should be more than just measuring; they should also be about comparing practice with agreed, appropriate, guidelines and procedures of care whenever available. Clinical audit is a dynamic process and the appropriateness of the standard may change in the light of new evidence. It may be necessary to carry out an audit before a standard is fully developed in order to explore the existence of a problem and the extent of it (Buckley 1997).

How to develop a standard. As discussed previously, standards need to based on the best available research evidence, rigorously derived clinical guidelines or consensus of 'expert' opinion. Standards of care must be drawn up in collaboration with a representative of all those who are involved with delivering the care under review, and, wherever appropriate, by a representative of those receiving the care, the consumer.

Practitioners, in particular midwives, need to be totally committed to the ethos of standard development by involving all the 'stakeholders' in this process. For example, the 'stakeholders' for a pregnant woman with diabetes should include the woman, general practitioner, diabetic liaison nurse, midwife, obstetrician, physician, dietitian, partner or other family members and paediatrician. From the outset, all representatives must understand the essential requirement that all standards developed must undergo continuous updating and refinement within an agreed time frame. In Chapter 6, Jenny Hall and Sue Hawkins provide an overview of the range of data sources which can inform the evidence base of standard development.

Some sources of data

- *Research information* – systematic reviews; literature searches, e.g. Medline, Cochrane Library, Cinhal, BIDS ISI data service; published data; contacting researchers in the field of interest.
- *Guidelines/recommendations* – national, regional and local.
- *Standards for practice* – national, regional and local.
- *Professional organizations* – Royal College of Midwives (RCM), Royal College of Obstetricians and Gynaecologists (RCOG), Royal College of Paediatrics and Child Health (RCPCH), Royal College of General Practitioners (RCGP).
- *Consumer groups* – National Childbirth Trust (NCT), Support Around Termination for Fetal Abnormalities (SATFA), Stillbirths and Neonatal

Death Society (SANDS), Miscarriage Society, Association for Improvements in Maternity Services (AIMS), Maternity Alliance, British Diabetic Association, British Epileptic Society.

Practical issues of undertaking audit and standard development for midwives

Midwives need to be prepared for their role as consumers and users of the audit process, if they are to participate in the delivery of quality maternity care. The following exercises explore some issues which need to be considered when planning or assessing audit proposals and standards.

Box 9.6 The audit process

1. Before you start, have you assessed the quality of evidence and the standards being used? Think about audits undertaken in your unit. Do you know who was involved, was it collaborative and multi-disciplinary, if not, do you know why not?
2. How often have you been asked to change practice as result of audit and not even known it was being conducted? Who is likely to create barriers to change? Have such people been included in the design phase? Have you set a date or some time aside to re-audit and evaluate practice in the future?

What to audit

Clinical audit is linked to ensuring that agreed standards of care are being achieved. Topics for audit can be generated from practitioners reflecting on aspects of care to problematic practice issues to structured collaborative group approaches. A number of units have established clinical audit groups or committees which should be approached before undertaking any aspect of an audit. It could be that the topic of interest to be explored is part of their annual agenda.

Examples of the most frequently audited topics undertaken by midwives

- Infant feeding – breastfeeding
- Perineal trauma
- Antenatal care – continuity of carer, frequency of visits
- Eating in labour
- Induction of labour
- Management of women who are RhD negative
- Caesarean section.

(Source: RCOG Clinical Audit Unit database 1998)

It is worthwhile checking the Trust's annual reports as there will be a section on audits undertaken in maternity care and gynaecology. The

---

Box 9.7   Some topics suitable for audit

Some of the Antenatal quality indicators from the PANDA Project (Vause & Maresh 1999)
- Women who are RhD negative – appropriate management during pregnancy i.e. antibody checks and sensitizing events
- Diagnosis of breech from 37 week gestation
- Number of antenatal visits
- Number of carers in antenatal period
- Continuity of carer.

Some quality indicators from the Prenatal Screening project (Wray & Maresh 1998)
- Pre-test information
- Local guidelines available
- Women's understanding of the purpose of tests undertaken
- Staff's perceptions of their training needs
- Giving back of results.

Breastfeeding
- Initiation and continuation rates
- Regular updating and regular training sessions are available for all staff who give advice to women.

Cross boundary care: organizational and communication issues
- Who takes responsibility?
- Clear lines of communication – access to lead professionals available.

---

clinical audit department is a useful resource and will have access to information in relation to audits past, present and possibly future initiatives. Box 9.7 shows suggestions for topics suitable for audit.

Who to audit

It is important at the outset to define clearly how many women, or cases, to involve in the audit. This is known as the *audit sample* or *audit population* (Campbell & Macfarlane 1994). This ensures that the standard developed is appropriate to the sample which is being evaluated. There is a temptation to collect extra data items 'while we are there … we may as well look at shoe size!' But what does this tell us?

When to audit

The notion of 'changes over time' is one which needs to be borne in mind, as a snap shot view of any aspect of care could lead to incorrect assumptions being made and unnecessary changes in care delivery. The data collected could be either retrospective or prospective. For example, a topical issue being explored is caesarean section rates. Such evaluations need to examine the rates over the past years (retrospective), and compare appropriately with current practice (prospective). Equally, it could be that, before introducing a change or new intervention, an audit prior to such changes is a valuable benchmark by which comparisons can be made.

Creating a culture for change

An essential component in the development of any clinical audit and quality initiative is the potential in the workplace for change. The results of clinical audit will require either a change in clinical practice or sustainability of practice. Therefore, issues of change management need to be carefully considered in the design and development stages. Although no easy undertaking, it is worth emphasizing that the potential to change clinical practice is facilitated by the feedback of audit information (Thomson et al 1998). It has been shown that information feedback is most likely to influence clinical practice if the information is presented close to the time of decision-making and the clinicians have previously agreed to review their practice (Mugford et al 1991). However, it needs to be recognized that a combination of strategies such as observation within one's own practice environment, multi-disciplinary and intersectoral audit initiatives which involve 'face to face' meetings, and discussions all influence patterns for change and feedback processes (Allery et al 1997). Strategies such as educational materials, conferences, reminders, written material, involvement of opinion leaders, primary care and patient mediated interventions need to be combined as methods for information feedback. In addition, for this feedback to be effective, it needs to be on-going, as the effects have been shown to decrease over time (Thomson et al 1998).

Initiating information feedback, changes and improvements may require practitioners to alter their attitude and agenda and create a culture of collaboration and co-operation. In other words, a team approach. As Berwick discusses;

'Great clinicians do not make great health care. Great clinicians interacting well with all of the other elements of the health care system make great health care' (adapted from Berwick 1997).

It could be argued that to improve the quality of health care does not necessarily require better professions or professionals, but better systems of work. This means interaction which achieves shared aims and sustains improved systems of working (Berwick 1997). In addition, clinical audit initiatives and standard development in maternity care need to focus on equity and the breaking down of professional barriers. This can be achieved by establishing committed collaborative working patterns, co-operation among professions and a team approach which recognizes the woman as a team member (Benbow et al 1997). A good communication system is also essential if practitioners in maternity care are to retain ownership of the development of clinical practice.

Box 9.8 North Staffordshire Hospital Trust ASQUAM (Achieving Sustainable Quality in Maternity)

A multi-professional project launched in 1995, aiming to produce evidence-based standards for use in pregnancy and childbirth. These standards incorporate targets in care in each chosen area. Progress is measured by cyclical audit and feedback to providers. Topics are generated from multi-disciplinary meetings which include 'user' representatives.

Some maternity units have clinical audit and standard setting groups or committees such as the North Staffordshire Hospital NHS Trust ASQUAM programme. This programme has developed criteria by which initiatives are assessed (see Box 9.8).

Involving women

Standards should be drawn up with input from users of local service, reflecting a diversity of backgrounds and needs (RCOG 1995a, 1995b). Pregnant women are often informed consumers of care, therefore their involvement in quality issues, in particular clinical audit and standard setting, cannot be over stated. In the last decade, maternity services have led the way on seeking the views of women for the processes of monitoring and improving the quality of care (Sitzia & Wood 1997). Women often prepare birth plans and are increasingly involved in decisions about the management of their pregnancy. Good audit projects will pay attention to consumer involvement and satisfaction. In support of this, the NHS Management Executive has funded work in developing patient/user involvement in clinical audit and this has emphasized the importance of finding ways of involving service users (Kelson 1995).

The dynamic role of audit in maternity care should not be under-valued. However, participation in the audit process over the years has been rather passive and examples of women's active involvement in the audit process are few (Morrell 1996). This is changing at a national level, where patient representatives are invited to contribute to national committees such as the Department of Health National Screening Committee, antenatal screening sub-group.

In planning and developing quality health care, in particular clinical audit, the involvement of women creates empowerment. Practitioners are learning the importance of this concept. This has been highlighted by the participation of consumer group representation on committees such as the Community Health Councils and Maternity Services Liaison Committees which, increasingly, are playing a major role in issues related to quality and standards of maternity practice.

CONCLUSION

For clinical audit and standard development to move forward, clear relationships should be developed with a focus on key issues such as clinical effectiveness, patient-focused care, multi-professional team working and practice development. These are all valuable for implementing the findings of research (Morrell 1996). A good communication system is also essential if practitioners in maternity care are to retain ownership of the development of clinical practice (Wray & Maresh 1997).

Clinical audit and standard development are at the heart of high quality health care. Together they are important tools in maintaining and developing this high level of care. They inform about the care being provided, they identify where change is necessary, and they help monitor the impact of those changes (Burnett & Winyard 1998). Midwives need to embrace the quality agenda, as accountable practitioners. The 'culture is right' with clinical governance, quality and clinical effectiveness being advocated as the basis by which health services will be judged in the future (Department of Health 1997). Midwives need to be prepared for their role as consumers and users of the audit process if they are to participate in the delivery of quality maternity care in whatever setting they practise.

FURTHER READING

The Report on the Confidential Enquiries into Maternal Deaths, HMSO. Published every 3 years, this assesses the cause of death, the management received, highlights substandard care and makes recommendations for future care. This is the longest running confidential enquiry in the world. A 'must read' for all those involved in maternity care.

Confidential Enquiries into Stillbirth and Death in Infancy, HMSO. Published annually, this enquiry gives the causes and incidence of deaths and assesses in more detail the management of a selection. These reports often highlight a particular issue, such as sudden infant death syndrome. A 'must read' for all those involved in maternity care and care of the newborn.

All NHS Executive and many Dept. of Health documents are available free of charge – ring the NHS Hotline on 0541 555 455

REFERENCES

Allery LA, Owen PA, Robling MR 'Why General Practitioners and Consultants Change their Clinical Practice: a critical incident study' *British Medical Journal* 1997; **314:** 870–874

Allison J 'Midwives Step Out of the Shadows' in Campbell R, Macfarlane A *Where to be Born? The debate and the evidence* Second edition Oxford: National Perinatal Epidemiology Unit; 1994

Batstone G, Edwards M 'Clinical Audit – how do we proceed?' *Southampton Medical Journal* 1994; **10:1:** 13–18

Benbow A, Semple D, Maresh M *Effective Procedures in Maternity Care Suitable for Audit.* London: Royal College of Obstetricians and Gynaecologists Press; 1997

Berwick DM 'Medical Associations: guilds or leaders?' *British Medical Journal* 1997; **314:** 1564–1565

Buckley ER *Delivering Quality in Midwifery* London: Baillière Tindall; 1997

Burnett AC, Winyard G 'Clinical Audit at the Heart of Clinical Effectiveness' *Journal of Quality in Clinical Practice* 1998; **18:** 3–19

Campbell R, Macfarlane A *Where to be Born? The debate and the evidence* (Second edition) Oxford: National Perinatal Epidemiology Unit; 1994

Department of Health *Working for Patients* London, HMSO; 1989

Department of Health *Changing Childbirth. The report of the expert maternity group* London, HMSO; 1993a

Department of Health *Clinical audit: meeting and improving standards in healthcare* London, Department of Health, 1993b

Department of Health *The New NHS – Modern, Dependable* White Paper London: Department of Health; 1997

Department of Health *A First Class Service – Quality in the new NHS* London: Department of Health; 1998a

Department of Health *Screening of pregnant women for hepatitis B and immunisation of babies at risk* HSC: 1998/127; 1998b

Dunn PM, McIlwaine G *Perinatal Audit – A Report Produced for the European Association of Perinatal Medicine* Carnforth: Parthenon Publishing Group; 1996

Gallant B, McLane A 'Outcome Criteria – a process for validation at unit level' *Journal of Nursing and Administration* 1979; **9:** 14

Hopkins A 'Clinical Audit: time for reappraisal?' *Journal of the Royal College of Physicians* 1996; **30(5):** 415–425

Kelson M *Consumer Involvement Initiatives in Clinical Audit and Outcomes.* London: College of Health; 1995 (*Copies available free of charge from Publication Unit, St Margaret's House, College of Health, 21 Old Ford Road, London E2 9PL.*)

Maresh M *Audit in Obstetrics and Gynaecology* Oxford: Blackwell Scientific Publications; 1994

Morrell C 'Clinical Audit Makes Progress in Care and Teamwork' *Nursing Times* 1996; **92(30):** 34–36

Moulder C *Miscarriage: Women's Experiences and Needs* Pandora Press; 1991

Mugford M, Banfield P, O-Hanlon M 'Effects of Feedback of Information on Clinical Practice: a review' *British Medical Journal* 1991; **303:** 398–402

RCOG *Organizational Standards for Maternity Services – the report of a joint working group* London, Royal College of Obstetricians and Gynaecologists Press; 1995a

RCOG *Communication Standards – Obstetrics, the report of a joint working group* London, Royal College of Obstetricians and Gynaecologists Press; 1995b

Sitzia J, Wood N 'Patient Satisfaction: a review of issues and concepts' *Social Science and Medicine* 1997; **45(12):** 1829–1843

Thomson MA, Oxman AD, Haynes RB et al in Neilson JP, Crowther CA, Hodnett ED, Hofmeyer GJ, Keirse MJNC *Pregnancy and Childbirth Module of The Cochrane Database of Systematic Reviews* Oxford: The Cochrane Library; The Cochrane Collaboration, Issue 1 Update Software; 1998

Vause S, Maresh M Indicators of quality of antenatal care: a pilot study *British Journal of Obstetrics and Gynaecology* 1999; **106:** 197–205

Wray J, Maresh M 'Multi-professional guidelines: Can we move beyond tribal boundaries?' *Quality in Health Care* 1997; **6:** 57–58

Wray J, Maresh M 'Prenatal screening audit' Poster, 28th British Congress of Obstetrics and Gynaecology *British Journal of Obstetrics and Gynaecology* 1998; **105(17):** 68

10

Education for best practice

M Rose Allen

KEY ISSUES

- Issues relating to midwives' accountability and the need to ensure best practice.
- The fundamental skills needed at pre-registration level.
- The structure and framework of continuing professional development.

- The need for partnership for best practice.
- The role of the midwifery educator.
- The importance of change management.
- Issues relating to health care trusts, statutory bodies, supervisors and managers.

INTRODUCTION

Midwives have to accommodate conventions, policies, procedures and guidelines, as well as women's wishes, into their everyday practice. Midwives also, like other health care professionals, have to account for their actions. They, therefore, need to develop strategies to ensure that not just safe but the best practice is offered to women, babies and their families. With the ever-increasing demands for evidence-based practice, employers and employees alike need to collaborate in endeavours to enhance such practice.

The structural foundations at national and regional levels to support evidence-based practice are only now developing. The government are planning to invest around £1 billion over the next 3 years in research activities. The National Institute for Clinical Excellence (NICE), Commission for Health Improvement (CHI) and Regional Research and Development Directorates are all part of their strategy. It appears from the White Paper for England, *Modern – Dependable* (Department of Health 1997), that implementing research in practice has at last been given the green light.

At a local level, health care trusts have an important role in supporting evidence-based practice, ranging from corporate policies to supporting individual midwives. The infrastructure of trusts needs to be developed further for the implementation of evidence-based practice to be carried out effectively. The process may be enhanced by the introduction of clinical governance. Some trusts already have active research portfolios and are collaborating to support staff development in enabling evidence-based practice, through, for example, providing local access to the Cochrane Library and employing practice-based development midwives to support and advise midwives on practice issues. Some of the strategies which facilitate midwives in their attempts to offer evidence-based practice need few resources. For example, employers are encouraging a culture of openness, where midwives are able to question and challenge practice. It is not always easy to challenge well established practices. Therefore a flexible, co-operative approach is essential if traditional practices are to be replaced by the best possible care.

Implementing best practice based on sound evidence needs excellent undergraduate and ongoing education, combined with partnerships between midwives and managers, and commitment, respect and tenacity on all sides.

ACCOUNTABILITY AND BEST PRACTICE

Evidence-based care can save lives; for example, the midwife who is familiar with the research on sleeping positions of infants and the relationship with Sudden Infant Death Syndrome (SIDS) can advise mothers on the best way to lay babies down in the cot to prevent this happening (Fleming et al 1996). Being accountable practitioners requires that midwives are educated to be able to provide evidence-based care, and that they continue to develop professionally throughout their professional careers.

Midwives should be aware that they are accountable for their own practice (UKCC 1998a). In case they are in any doubt, they are reminded that '... the standard of practice in the delivery of midwifery care shall be that which is acceptable in the context of *current knowledge and clinical developments ...*' (UKCC 1994).

Within *post-registration and practice* (PREP) requirements, nurses, midwives and health visitors need to provide evidence every 3 years that they are up-to-date (UKCC 1997a). This is a requirement for continued practice. Some midwives, in addition to this, have to provide evidence of completing a statutory refresher course every 5 years (UKCC 1997b). The United Kingdom Central Council for nursing, midwifery and health visiting (UKCC) continues to inform and advise professionals of the issues relating to PREP. The UKCC (1997b) have also produced specific information for midwives which gives examples of what they need to do to meet statutory requirements. Some midwives remain rather perplexed, as they have difficulty in assimilating yet another change. However, midwives have a valuable resource in the form of their supervisors who are well versed in the statutory requirements. Issues concerning registration, maintenance of and return to practice affect all practising midwives. Midwives should make it their business, as accountable practitioners, to be well informed.

Midwives also know that while pre-registration education provides some knowledge and skills, it is necessary for them to enhance their skills and acquire new knowledge to be sure that they are delivering, not only safe, but best care. It is essential that midwives constantly reflect, question and challenge practice. Therefore, they must be knowledgeable about current evidence derived from good research, as well as other issues which affect how they offer care, in its broadest sense. This requires not only excellent pre-registration education, but also effective continuing education and training.

Pre-registration education

Since 1996, all midwifery education in England has been based in universities. There is a range of programmes, including:

- 3-year degree programmes
- 3-year diploma programmes
- 18-month degree programmes for qualified nurses
- 18-month diploma programmes for qualified nurses
- Some 4-year degree programmes which are unlikely to continue.

All of these programmes lead to registration as a midwife on part 10 of the UKCC register. The entry requirements for the various programmes are different. The English National Board (ENB) require a minimum of five general certificates of education or equivalent, including English and a science subject, all of which must be grade C or above. Some universities ask for evidence of advanced levels of general knowledge, whilst others specify certain subjects.

The recent ENB (1998a) guidelines for pre-registration midwifery pro-grammes advise that, on completion of the programme, midwives must be able to base their practice on the best available evidence. Pre-registration programmes have a range of ways of providing academic input and clinical experience. It is crucial that the programmes are planned to allow students to fully integrate theory and practice, so that they can see the benefits of their academic education in the practice setting. Half of the student's experience is spent in the practice setting; this means that a close partnership between education and practice is essential. To assess if students can receive the appropriate experiences, clinical as well as educational audits should be undertaken at regular intervals.

Midwifery lecturers should be 'linked' with clinical areas to support the students and staff in the provision of best care. Clinical staff should be encouraged to communicate with lecturers and vice versa, to question what students are being taught regarding research and best care. 'Triad' meetings between the midwife mentor, student and midwifery lecturer should take place, to ensure the students and their clinical mentors know about good practices, and that the lecturer understands the clinical problems and experiences the student is encountering. Tutorials and seminar sessions in practice are another means whereby students learn more about evidence-based care. Throughout the programme of study, students should keep records of their experiences in the form of a portfolio and/or a reflective diary, and they should be encouraged to question whether best practice is being provided in light of the current evidence.

Students undertake a range of assessments during their programme of study, in a variety of settings. They have to pass assessments at different levels. They are tested on their ability to search and analyse critically the evidence on which they and others base their care, and should also be assessed on their ability to question the value of the findings. They should be assessed on their interpersonal skills and, in particular, be able to assess themselves.

Good interpersonal skills are essential, as they help newly qualified midwives to be accepted and valued as team members. Assessment should also include the development and maintenance of partnerships with women and their families. A team member who continues to develop, who is knowledgeable about current evidence and is able to articulate in a thoughtful manner why certain practices should be changed to facilitate best care, is a valuable asset for the profession. As good team members, midwives are more likely to be listened to by their peers and their senior colleagues.

Post-registration education – lifelong learning

Many midwives have been educated on programmes which have provided them with the analytical skills needed to practise evidence-based care. Nevertheless some have not, and all midwives need ongoing education – lifelong learning as it is now called.

Oakley & Houd (1990) have described midwifery practice in the past as being like a jigsaw. Individuals try to fit together politics and economics, as well as secular and religious aspects, to bring about good. These pieces of the jigsaw are still relevant for today's midwifery practitioners, as they try to offer safe care, in addition to dealing with issues arising from developing empirical evidence, science, technology and management structures and processes across the NHS.

As science and health technology develop, new discoveries are made which provide evidence that may be used to improve care. To ensure that up-to-date evidence-based care is offered to women and their babies, midwives need to have access to scientific and technological information through effective study programmes on a regular basis. As with most decisions that are made in the NHS, however, the midwife's development is influenced by efficiency savings and cost effectiveness, as well as clients' needs. It will be interesting to monitor whether the call for a statutory instrument to measure clinical effectiveness, recommended in the White Paper for the NHS in England (Department of Health 1997), will influence the support midwives obtain from employers when attempting to update themselves.

A programme of study cannot, on its own, ensure learning and best practice. For example, factors such as individual motivation, confidence and responsibility affect a professional's personal learning. The needs and wants of midwives do not always match the programme or service outcomes, and effective resourcing in relation to time, monies and meaningful communication about continuing development are not always addressed. These issues are just a few highlighted by writers on professional education (McClellend 1970, Study & Hunt 1980, Crotty 1984, Mander 1986, Rogers & Lawrence 1987, Hack 1987, Brown 1988, Clarke & Rees 1988, Hewitt 1991, Nolan et al 1995, Pope et al 1996).

Nevertheless, it is argued that continuing professional development for nurses, midwives and health visitors is essential (Brown 1988, Whiteley 1989, Hewitt 1991, Nolan et al 1995, Pope et al 1996). The purpose of continuing professional development is to enhance the knowledge and skills of health care professionals, to inform practice and, ultimately, to maintain and enhance standards to facilitate safe and best care. It is crucial, therefore, to support professional development. Although there is an abundance of theoretical literature on this subject, Nolan et al (1995) suggest that there is insufficient empirical information or research about the best way to do it. Professional opinions suggest, however, that the changes in the management and organization of the NHS and higher education, including the purchaser–provider split and full course cost recovery, have thwarted professional development.

In some instances the business-like basis on which the NHS now operates appears at odds with health care professionals' aspirations for development, as the organization's goals take priority. The clinical perspective of what the service needs, for example an adequate number of midwives on duty caring for women (not on study leave), may also inhibit professional development. Indeed, Nolan et al (1995) and Pope et al (1996) identified a number of barriers to continuing professional education which include staff shortages, time and finance. Nolan et al (1995) recognize that professionals can become demotivated and suggest that the values and beliefs of the organization have to endorse development positively for their employees. This would seem particularly important if employers value an up-to-date workforce which is able to provide evidence-based care. The majority of trusts have mission statements and objectives that imply that they support professional development and endeavour to formulate strategies to support these.

The lack of adequate resources to support professional development appears to compound the difficulties that midwives experience in their endeavours to develop professionally (Pansini-Murrell 1994, Nolan et al 1995, Pope et al 1998). It appears that the increase in demand from health care professionals for effective resourcing of development programmes is unlikely to be met in the future, essentially because the resourcing of such programmes is not always seen as a priority. It could even be suggested that professional development may become another 'Cinderella' of the health service. In extreme cases, some midwives might argue that their development is obstructed. In the short term, lack of professional development may lead to midwives having limited current knowledge to support evidence-based practice. In the long term, this lack of development may contribute to sub-standard care or malpractice. Considering all these issues, it has never been so important for midwives to use, and to be able to use, current evidence when offering care to their clients, in order that the best, as well as a safe, standard of care is achieved.

Investing in best practice

The complexities that face midwives regarding professional development appear to be never-ending. Nevertheless, it is their responsibility to ensure they remain up-to-date to offer best, as well as safe, care to mothers, babies and their families. To meet the professional development needs of midwives locally, many trusts are investing resources in professional development programmes. Many have expanded their own training departments to facilitate staff development. Some, for example, have employed professionals with a specific remit to enhance evidence-based practice in posts such as *Lecturer/Practitioner*, *Project Officer*, *Research/Practice Development Midwife* and *Research Midwife*. In addition, some trusts have agreed strategies which encourage joint appointments between service and academic institutions to secure best practice through research. Indeed, at regional and district levels, some trusts are working in partnership with research and development departments to bid for research fellowship awards which, as well as other benefits, facilitate professional development, address practice issues and, ultimately, may enhance care. Although midwives can take responsibility for their own professional development, they need support from managers and colleagues to be able to provide best care.

At a national level, effective strategies to support this must be devised between the Department of Health, NHS Executive and statutory bodies. These should then be cascaded down to Health Authorities, Primary Care Groups and Trusts. Such developments are described in the White Paper (Department of Health 1997). Clinical governance may enhance such collaboration once it is introduced in 1999.

Supervisors of midwives also have an important role to play in ensuring best practice and, therefore, should aim to support midwives in developing their knowledge of evidence derived from research. The supervisory and practice review interviews used by supervisors and managers to assess midwives' practice needs is one way of assisting midwives in planning for their practice development.

There is no doubt, midwives need to keep up to date through education and training to offer safe care which is evidence-based, but this often requires an act of juggling the jigsaw pieces by practising midwives until they all fit.

Post-registration legislation has had, and will continue to have, far-reaching effects on health professionals who wish to continue to practise. Indeed, the UKCC and the ENB are presently consulting on a higher level of practice which will be based upon national standards of clinical competence, the outcome of which may also result in further legislation. Presently, health care professionals, including midwives, need to provide evidence that they are up-to-date in their area of practice on a 3 yearly basis. If employers, employees, educational institutes and statutory bodies are prepared to work together, with a shared vision to inform their aims and objectives, successful professional development programmes should not be too difficult for midwives to achieve.

Structure for supporting continuing professional development

In 1989 the ENB undertook a project to investigate how health care professionals could best meet the needs of their clients. The phrase 'Quality Education for Quality Care' was established. The outcome of this project was a comprehensive, flexible, coherent framework for professional educational developments. This framework provided qualified professionals with the opportunity to acquire both academic credits and professional expertise. Its philosophy encouraged a partnership between educators and service managers where values could be shared to ultimately enhance safe care (ENB 1991a). The Framework and Higher Award recognize experience and allow for accumulation and transfer of academic credits. Professionals who obtain 120 credits at level 3 (honours degree level) and achieve the Ten Key Characteristics (ENB 1991b), acquire both academic and professional recognition. These ten key characteristics include clinical skills, quality care and research. The ENB (1998b) consultation document on continuing professional education has retained the principles of these ten key characteristics (see Box 10.1).

Although this was an innovative approach, incorporating modularization and credit accumulation, it appears to have lost its appeal for some midwives. The modules can be costly, and attending the taught programmes in addition to the time spent studying and writing assignments has proved to be too demanding for many. Nevertheless, programmes do help midwives to acquire the necessary skills to understand what evidence

Box 10.1 10 key characteristics

Midwives should show:

1. The ability to exercise professional accountability and responsibility, reflected in the degree to which the practitioner uses professional skills, knowledge and expertise in changing environments, across professional boundaries, and in unfamiliar situations.
2. Specialist skills, knowledge and expertise in the practice area where working, including a deeper and broader understanding of client/patient health needs, within the context of changing health care provision.
3. The ability to use research to plan, implement and evaluate concepts and strategies leading to improvements in care.
4. Team working, including multi-professional team working, in which the leadership role changes in response to changing client needs, team leadership and team building skills to organize the delivery of care.
5. The ability to develop and use flexible and innovative approaches to practice appropriate to the needs of the client/patient or group in line with the goals of the health service and the employing authority.
6. Understanding and use of health promotion and preventative policies and strategies.
7. The ability to facilitate and assess the professional and other developments of all for whom responsible, including, where appropriate, learners and to act as a role model of professional practice.
8. The ability to take informed decisions about the allocation of resources for the benefit of individual clients and the client group with whom working.
9. The ability to evaluate quality of care delivered as an on-going and cumulative process.
10. The ability to facilitate, initiate, manage and evaluate change in practice to improve quality of care.

(ENB 1991b)

is acceptable for best practice. For example, midwives who undertake research modules are assessed on their ability to describe, discuss, and appraise research. Some modules require midwives to analyse research critically, while others require them to carry out research in practice. However, hot on the heels of the Framework and Higher Award, came the statutory instrument for Post-Registration and Practice (PREP).

Post-registration education and practice (PREP)

In 1990 the UKCC commissioned a project on post-registration education. Almost 28,000 people returned a prepaid postcard which was sent out by the project group. A further 1,338 responses were received in full following consultation. The main focus of the project was concerned with providing a coherent pattern of education for professionals to ensure safe practice. For midwives, PREP is concerned with professional development in order to maintain and improve standards of care.

PREP enables midwives to embrace a flexible, pragmatic approach to learning. The study activities must be equivalent to 5 days (at least 35 hours of professional development) every 3 years, in order to remain on the professional register.

In addition to suggesting conferences and courses to facilitate a safe standard of care, the UKCC (1997a) advises professionals that they may undertake individual and/or group activities; these include:

- literature searches
- research projects
- seminar presentations
- visits to inform practice.

Midwives, like other health care professionals, are advised by the UKCC (1997a) to keep a professional portfolio. The portfolio should provide evidence that the midwife is up-to-date in their area of practice. Brown (1992) has two definitions relating to professional portfolios which are worth remembering.

Professional portfolio

'A private collection of evidence which demonstrates learning and application to professional practice.'

Personal profile

'Selected evidence from the portfolio which demonstrates learning for a specific purpose' (Brown 1992).

The UKCC (1997a) advises professionals to follow six stages to facilitate their maintenance of the portfolio and to enable relevant professional development. They are:

1. *Reflection*
2. *Objective setting*
3. *Action planning*
4. *Implementation of plans*
5. *Evaluation*
6. *Recording learning outcomes.*

Although these profiles will be self-verified, a formal audit of profiles will commence on the 1st of April 2001. In the meantime, a pilot study is being undertaken to establish an effective evaluation system (UKCC 1998b).

The NHS Executive (1998) has published an information pack for nurses, midwives and health visitors to support effective practice, which will also be suitable for PREP and which includes information to support evidence-based practice. This pack includes information on:

- clinical effectiveness
- searching and critically appraising the literature

- preparation, designing and conducting clinical audit
- preparing a research proposal and designing a research study
- changing clinical practice
- writing and publishing.

The UKCC's (1998c) consultation document on a Higher Level of Practice, if accepted, will further influence professional development.

The role of midwifery educators in supporting evidence-based practice

As midwifery moves to an all-graduate profession, as suggested by the Standing Nursing and Midwifery Advisory Committee (Department of Health 1998), it may become easier for some midwives to critically evaluate the evidence on which they base their practice. However, presently there are many who need support and encouragement in a safe environment to implement practices from effective evidence. Midwifery educators, therefore, have an important role in assisting these midwives in becoming more critical, through their clinical link and teaching roles. Supporting and encouraging midwives to evaluate their practice is a vital skill that clinical link midwife lecturers must possess. The educators who sit in 'ivory towers' and pronounce words of wisdom will rarely secure midwives' attention long enough to begin to support their understanding of a complex and sometimes common sense appraisal of research. They, therefore, will be unable to bridge the gap between research and practice.

The practical, applied approach relevant to the midwives' practice must be the key to understanding. Educationalists should ensure that the learning process is meaningful and fulfilling. Stocking (1993) quite rightly argues that research needs to be in touch with reality. Not only has it to be 'in touch' but for changes to occur in practice, research must be disseminated. It must 'connect' significantly with every day practice and be used as the basis by educators to facilitate learning.

Supporting change for best care

Midwives are often enthusiastic and motivated, but they have been involved in many changes in the past decade and the commitment to do things differently is not always easy to foster, especially if the reasoning does not appear to make sense. Therefore, midwives, like other health care professionals, must be convinced that change is necessary, not just for the sake of change, but to make practice more effective. To gain their trust, midwives need to be valued as both individuals and experts.

While this chapter does not intend to debate the benefits of change strategies, it is important to note they are in important factor if new or different

---

Box 10.2 Thinking about change

Think about the process of introducing change within your unit or team. By yourself or in a group, think about the following statements and questions. How might they be answered for your area of practice?

1. People need to feel secure. (*Do you have any evidence that this is so?*)
2. Partnerships need to be formed between everyone who is involved in care. (*Do you know how cohesive these partnerships are?*)
3. The organization needs to value research. (*What resources are available at the bedside for this to be effective?*)
4. Resources need to be available, but not necessarily in abundance. (*How do you know that resources are being used appropriately?*)

---

approaches to care are to be accommodated effectively into the everyday practice of the midwife. Of course, certain things have to be in place before any change can take place (see Box 10.2).

It is important that leaders of change have enthusiasm and are respected by their colleagues and peers, as it can be a labour of love to try to implement something new when old practices seem to be working extremely well.

We all need to recognize that the pursuit of the application of evidence to support best practice in midwifery and other areas of practice takes time. Application of research findings must be seen as meaningful, and effective discussion must take place to facilitate understanding, acceptance and application. Rejection of inappropriate change must be considered as a viable option. Finally an audit of practice should take place on a regular basis to ensure best care is not just being talked about but actually delivered.

Practical stages to facilitate change should include:

- *Discussion*
- *Understanding*
- *Connection*
- *Rejection*
- *Application*
- *Audit.*

Of course, fundamental to any change is a careful exploration of the practice, to ensure that the change being proposed is based in the best possible evidence!

CONCLUSION

Midwives work in a very demanding profession which, because of its very nature, requires a continued commitment to providing best care. Midwives need to develop skills in supporting evidence-based practice, including critical appraisal, information technology awareness, communication skills and change management. In order for this to be successful, strategies are needed, particularly collaboration between the NHS Executive, Department of Health, statutory bodies, health authorities, trusts, local supervising authorities and professional associations. In addition, there need to be sufficient resources and an enthusiasm and willingness from midwives, supervisors and employers and midwifery leaders to support opportunities for developing the knowledge and skills of midwives which are essential in developing evidence-based care.

FURTHER READING

NHS Executive *Achieving Effective Practice: A Clinical Effectiveness and Research Information Pack for Nurses, Midwives and Health Visitors* London: DoH; 1998
This information pack guides the practitioner through ten stages to achieve clinical effectiveness. The material includes information on searching and critically appraising the literature; material on clinical audit and changing clinical practice is also included. Section 8 and 9 of the information pack focuses upon designing studies and preparing a research proposal. The final section provides information on writing and publishing on clinical effectiveness.
Polit D F, Hungler B P *Essentials of Nursing Research* Lippincot; 1997
This comprehensive research text explores and explains research methods, and the utilization of research.
UKCC *Midwives' Refresher Courses and PREP* UKCC; 1997
This booklet seeks to clarify the transitional arrangements for midwives regarding refresher courses and PREP

REFERENCES

Brown LA 'Maintaining Professional Practice – Is Continuing Education a Cure or Merely a Tonic?' *Nurse Education Today* 1988; **8(5):** 251–257
Brown RA *Portfolio Development and Profiling for Nurses* Lancaster: Quay Publishing; 1992
Clarke J, Rees C 'The Midwife and Continuing Education' *Midwives Chronicle* 1988(Sept); 288–290
Crotty M 'Continuing Education; a Practice Experience' *Nurse Education Today* 1984; **4(1):** 20–21
Department of Health *The New NHS – Modern, Dependable* London: Department of Health; 1997
Department of Health *Midwifery: Delivering Our Future* Report by the Standing Nursing and Midwifery Advisory Committee London: Department of Health; 1998
English National Board *Framework for Continuing Professional Education for Nurses Midwives and Health Visitors* guide to implementation, London: ENB; 1991a
English National Board *Framework for Continuing Professional Education for Nurses Midwives and Health Visitors* guide to implementation summary card 1, London: ENB; 1991b
English National Board *Creating Lifelong Learners* London: ENB; 1998a
English National Board *Consultation on the Board's revised Continuing Professional Education Framework encompassing all post-registration studies programmes,* London: ENB; 1998b
Fleming PJ, Blair PS, Bacon C, Bensley D, Smith I, Taylor E, Berry J, Golding J, Tripp J 'Environments of Infants During Sleep and Risk of the Sudden Infant Death Syndrome: Results of 1993–5 Case-Control Study for Confidential Enquiry into Stillbirths and Deaths of Infants' *British Medical Journal* 1996; **313:** 191–194
Hack KA 'Predicting Success in Professional Courses' *Midwife Health Visitor and Community Nurse* 1987; **23(1):** 6–9

Hewitt G 'Enriching Lessons' *Nursing Times* 1991; **87(47):** 32–34

McClellend DC *The Achieving Society* London: Macmillan; 1970

McCrea H 'Motivation of Continuing Education' *Midwifery* 1989; **5:** 134–145

Mander R 'Refresher Courses – Unfilled Potential?' *Midwives Chronicle* 1986(Feb); 39–41

Nolan M, Glynn Owens R, Nolan J 'Continuing Professional Education: identifying the characteristics of an effective system' *Journal of Advanced Nursing* 1995; **2(1):** 551–560

NHS Executive *Achieving Effective Practice* Department of Health; 1998

Oakley A, Houd S *Helpers in Childbirth; Midwifery Today* New York: Taylor Francis; 1990

Pansini-Murrell J 'Is Continuing Education Dividing the Professional?' *British Journal of Midwifery*, 1994; **2(5):** 227–230

Pope R, Cooney L, Graham L, Holliday M, Patel S *Identification of the Changing Educational Needs of Midwives in Developing New Dimensions of Care in a Variety of Settings and the Development of an Educational Package to Meet these Needs* London: ENB; 1996

Pope R, Cooney L, Graham L, Holliday M, Patel S 'Aspects of Care 5: the continuing educational need of midwives' *British Journal of Midwifery* 1998; **6(4)**

Rogers J, Lawrence J *Continuing Professional Education for Nurses, Midwives and Health Visitors*, Peterborough: Ashdale Press in collaboration with Austin Cornish; 1987

Stocking B 'Implementing the Findings in Effective Care in Pregnancy and Childbirth in UK' *Milbank Quarterly* 1993; **71(3):** 497–521

Study S, Hunt S 'A Computerised Survey of Learning Needs' *Nursing Times* 1980(19 June); 1084–1086

UKCC *Midwives Code of Practice*, London: UKCC; 1994

UKCC *PREP and You*, London: UKCC; 1997a

UKCC *Midwives' Refresher Courses and PREP*, London: UKCC; 1997b

UKCC *Midwives Rules and Code of Practice*, London: UKCC; 1998a

UKCC *Register No 23*, London: UKCC; 1998b

UKCC *A Higher Level of Practice* (consultation document) London: UKCC; 1998c

Whiteley SJ (1989) 'The Construction of an Evaluative model for use in Conjunction with Continuing Education in the Nursing Profession' Unpublished PhD Thesis CNAA Queen Margaret College Edinburgh, Cited in Nolan et al; 1995

11

The reality of evidence-based practice in midwifery

Sue Proctor and Mary Renfrew

KEY ISSUES

- Focus group of practising midwives discussing their experiences of using research in clinical practice
- Factors considered to be helpful or unhelpful in developing evidence-based practice are identified
- Ways of strengthening the links between research and practice are suggested.

'I think if midwives want to become autonomous practitioners then they need to have research ... and have good rationale for their care with research'

Student midwife

INTRODUCTION

On the whole, midwives are agreed about the importance of using research evidence to inform practice. Many are also aware and have experiences which suggest that this is not an easy process. We wanted to discover more about the reality of using evidence in practice and arranged a discussion group of six midwives from various backgrounds and with different experiences. The participants included student midwives, and qualified midwives who worked in hospital and community settings. All contributed to the discussion and their opinions, experiences and suggestions are presented in this chapter.

Many issues were raised by the group, and overall, they expressed very positive attitudes to the use of research in developing practice. They did, however, identify barriers to the implementation of research in practice, but offered a range of ideas and suggestions as to how these could be addressed. Their discussion identified issues for midwives to consider, whether they are based in clinical practice, education, research or management. Some issues emerged which related to the way research is presented in professional journals, and to the way it is perceived by the profession. Differences in the way the midwives had learnt about research and how they expected to use it were apparent, especially between the students and more experienced midwives.

They discussed how the relationship of research to practice had changed over recent years and spoke of a range of important issues which may influence the future of midwifery and the continued development of evidence-based practice.

Their thoughts and perceptions are presented according to the themes we feel have emerged from listening to them and reading through the transcription of their discussion. They identified a range of factors believed to influence the use of evidence in current practice, either positively or negatively, and made suggestions about how some key problems might be addressed. In addition, some important issues around the future of research and its relationship to the unique role of the midwife were also discussed. These raise important points that will stimulate wider discussion within the profession. Some of these issues are developed further in the concluding chapter.

FACTORS WHICH INFLUENCE THE USE OF EVIDENCE IN MIDWIFERY

A lengthy discussion about the issues which participants felt to be helpful or unhelpful in implementing evidence in practice identified a range of diverse factors. Generally, the discussion was positive and participants often presented reasoned arguments, trying to understand why barriers to the use of research existed. Often they looked for ways to improve and develop practice, and showed a mutual respect for colleagues who felt challenged, even threatened, by the existence of the 'evidence-based culture'.

Factors felt to be unhelpful

Five main themes emerged from the discussion of factors felt to be unhelpful in developing evidence-based practice:

1. lack of support to change practice
2. the strength of midwives' beliefs in tradition and experience as a basis for practice
3. increasingly weak links between education and clinical practice
4. the influence of organizational culture/professional socialization
5. lack of skills in research appraisal.

Lack of support to change practice

The midwives spoke a great deal about the importance of being supported in clinical decision-making. This included support from peers, managers, medical staff and, particularly for students, lecturers. They also mentioned the sometimes negative influence of local policies which acted as a barrier to change,

'I think there was a piece of research that came out about using Cetrimide to clean someone before a vaginal examination and I know Hospital X stopped using it and began using tap water because it was found to be as effective ... although Hospital Y's staff read the piece of research and it seemed that it was conclusive, none of the midwives would change because their policy said 'clean with Cetrimide' and until that was changed, they wouldn't do it.'

Strength of midwives' beliefs in tradition

Factors such as 'resistance to change' and 'negative attitudes' are often cited as barriers to the implementation of research among health care professions. In this group, the midwives and students acknowledged this as an issue, but also reflected on the reasons why some midwives were reluctant to change their practice.

'Being emotionally involved in caring about our work makes it very hard for us to process information ... I think it's part of why some experienced midwives who have been doing something one way for years simply say, "I don't care, I'm not going to change". – You can imagine why they might say that if they feel very strongly that they've been doing the best thing for years.'

'It must be hard if you think you are doing the best thing for somebody and you've been doing it that way for years and never seen anybody come to any harm. Suddenly some young upstart comes along and says, "well I've read in so and so that you do it this way."'

There was recognition of the valuable contribution of experienced midwives. Participants' comments suggested a mutual respect and a desire to learn from each other in working towards improving the care for women and babies:

'... people always do things because they've always done it that way ... I think sometimes we're trying to throw the baby out with the bath water and we should be helping those practitioners to find out why they are doing that and why it always works, so you are not throwing out good things ... Some of these things do work and not everything that we do or have done in the past isn't any good just because there isn't any research to back it up. Perhaps if we went out there and looked for it we would find the evidence.'

'You know there are lots of really good things that people are doing and continue to do, but if you asked them which article they read it in or which piece of research they read that told them they can do that, they probably couldn't tell you, but it is not that it isn't good.'

Increasingly weak links between education and clinical practice

The group discussed changes in midwifery education and its relationship with practice since moving into the university setting. Among the senior midwives, there was much criticism of lecturers and their role in the clinical area.

'The midwifery tutors move into Higher Education then they seem to vanish from the face of the earth and the real dilemma appears because we've lost touch … They lost touch with the day-to-day practical issues of midwifery practice and I think the practising midwives lost trust in them to some extent.'

'There is still a core group of staff who are working in Higher Education institutions and they are not changing, they are not moving into the clinical arena …'

A fragmentation in the profession was observed by one midwife, who felt that differing perceptions among educators, clinicians and researchers was divisive and, in some cases, very damaging.

'I think the difficulty is, or has been and probably will be, that educators, practitioners and researchers, – all three of us – within any sphere of practice you've got your own language. You've got your own way of seeing things and doing things and there are no little footpaths across these little crevices which in some cases, aren't crevices – they're great big gorges.'

The group felt that greater integration between clinical and educational roles was needed. In addition, increased involvement of clinical midwives in an educating role.

'We certainly need more integration of roles between research and practice and practitioner–lecturer roles. I'd like to see more opportunities for clinicians to go out and delve into lots of different areas.'

'One way would be to try and involve practitioners at the grass roots level who are providing care on a one-to-one basis.'

The influence of organizational culture/professional socialization

The influence of local policy on the utilization of research evidence in practice was highlighted. The impact on local 'ways of working' was also identified, such as feeling obliged to 'clear the labour ward' before the arrival of the new shift. The group spoke of the influence of socialization into the culture of a particular unit, almost without realizing it.

'It's not 'cos people don't want to change, I think they are willing to change and they are aware that things need to be changed. It's the practicality of it. You get into a routine which is the norm and you have to do A, B and C and it has to be done by 3.00, and if it's not done then you get into trouble.'

'You just get socialized into where you are working, into the culture of the organization, into *that* way of doing things. You can see that it is just like a self perpetuating cycle when you look at labour ward midwives up and down the country how they are sort of labelled.'

Lack of skills in research appraisal

The lack of ability to assess the quality of a published research paper was identified by the group. They felt that many midwives did not possess these skills and, in cases where they wanted to change practice or go to their manager with an idea, this weakness prevented them from moving forward.

'If you haven't ever looked at research, you don't know how to analyse it. You think, well, how do I know if it's a good piece of research or not?'

'When you read a piece of research and you don't have knowledge of the research process, you are kind of held back a bit because you don't know if it is a good or bad piece of research, and whether you can actually bring it to your manager and say, "look at this".'

It was recognized that the ability to critically appraise research was only one element in the implementation of change, that the need for a desire to change and support from colleagues and the clinical manager were also crucial.

'It's not just being able to critically evaluate a piece of research, it's about how to implement that through managing the change within the clinical environment.'

An encouraging factor about the discussion on unhelpful factors was that the group did not focus only on negative issues or problems. They showed a great deal of motivation and determination in their desire to understand these issues, why they have developed and ways to address them.

Factors felt to be helpful

Three main themes emerged which related to factors that the group felt were helpful in enabling the implementation of research evidence into practice:

1. confidence and ability to manage change
2. opportunities to share information
3. support throughout the process.

Confidence and ability to manage change

The issue of managing change was linked closely to comments around support from clinical managers in the introduction of research findings to practice. The group discussed the importance of responding appropriately when a need to alter practice was identified. They also spoke of the need to recognize, as a manager, that change can be threatening and can generate resistance. One has to be careful about how the process is managed to minimize such risks.

'I think to generate change you need people in there who can manage the change. You need to be able to do that from the bottom up, rather than inflict something on staff through policy, which will stay for years without any adaptation ...'

'It is quite easy to be labelled as a trouble maker, but I think there are ways to try and change things. There are ways of saying things and doing things to try and get people on your side, rather than against you. It is certainly extremely difficult as a student midwife to challenge the practice of somebody with lots of years' experience.'

Opportunities to share information

The participants spoke at length of the value of sharing information. In the various units where they practised, there was a range of examples of such activity. Opportunities for information exchange were felt to be beneficial in developing ownership of change among midwives, as an example of working with and learning from medical colleagues and, generally, as a non-threatening way of challenging practice. Examples of different approaches to sharing information, which were felt to be helpful included:

'It is so important for midwives and medical staff to share experiences and that includes *critical incident reporting forums, perinatal mortality meetings* ... and we have *feedback and reflection forms* for midwives to complete so the midwives can share the information that they received on a particular study event.'

'Usually we do *debates between the doctors and midwives*. We've done one on ARM and basically we debated for ARM and we put the doctors on the spot to debate against it. It was really good because you get both sides of the coin. You can see where they are coming from and, equally, they can see our point of view.'

'Through *midwives identifying their special interests and using reflection*, being given the opportunity to set up sessions, to go out and find the evidence and share the knowledge with people in their own practice area. If you can do that you can convince your manager that this is the way forward, this is the evidence ...'

'It's really important to have *reflective groups*, or just to sit down with coffee and have a chat and bring what you've read, do that *on a regular basis*. People need to think it is as valuable as giving time to women, because it can improve your care to all the women that you look after.'

Support throughout the process

The importance of support was identified as a common theme throughout the discussion. It was an issue of relevance to students and experienced midwives. Mentorship, preceptorship and clinical supervision were all identified as extremely valuable in enabling midwives learn and develop their practice. Support from colleagues was also identified – from midwives, doctors and other professions. There was clear recognition that midwives could not implement changes individually but needed commitment from the team.

'If you've got somebody who is supporting you, whether that's a mentor if you're a student or a preceptor if you're newly qualified or a supervisor, then I think that makes you more likely to want to try and implement things – if you've got a supportive environment.'

'You need a system that provides a framework which is supportive. In midwifery we have supervision of midwives which is ideal for getting people on board with evidence-based practice and to change their old practice ... It is now used to develop proactive support for midwives, not just in critical incidents in their day-to-day activity, but particularly with professional development and other opportunities.'

The support required by newly qualified staff was specifically identified. It was felt that this group of midwives had a vast amount of theoretical knowledge, and a high level of motivation. Support through their transition to experienced midwife was important to harness this enthusiasm, help them gain the experience they lacked, and use their theoretical knowledge effectively.

'It's important, especially for newly qualified midwives, to have a lot of support because you are actually quite motivated when you start a new job and, if you've got support, you'll keep motivated ...'

Issues of recruitment and retention of such staff were also raised and support was felt to be a key component in encouraging keen midwives to stay in the profession.

An additional issue was identified in relation to support – it is important to give positive, honest feedback and to acknowledge when midwives had changed their practice for the better, particularly when change had been threatening.

'It has been a big transformation for a lot of midwives, but they have risen to the challenge. I would have to admire them for doing that. For me, what's very rewarding is when a midwife does change practice so that it is evidence based.'

ISSUES FOR DEBATE

Two key issues emerged from the discussion which were felt to have an important impact on the understanding and utilization of research evidence in clinical practice. These were closely integrated and related to perceptions – of the role of the midwife and the image of research in midwifery.

Midwifery – art or science?

The group debated how midwives had to combine a nurturing role, which they saw in the context of interpersonal skills and individualized care of women, with a scientific, more objective role in clinical activity and in the conduct and application of research. By some of the participants, these elements were felt to be at odds with one another. It was felt that the caring, nurturing part of the midwifery role was undervalued in much published research. Further, that it was not appreciated by other professionals.

'Others from outside the midwifery arena don't see nurturing and science as being merged. I think they see science as the way we should be going and nurturing; well to me, the nurturing bit is actually looked down upon, whereas I think it is the most important bit. Sometimes by going towards the scientific bit we are losing the most important part of our role.'

'It's not just midwifery, it's everything and … even as a student and as a staff nurse, the majority of people are quite receptive to the fact that everything has to be evidence-based. But basically, fundamentally, why we came into this profession, is because we are carers.'

This led to a discussion about the origins of much research in midwifery, that often research questions arose from a desire to change practice, to improve women's experiences of childbirth. Much research in midwifery is driven by the emotional involvement and care felt by midwives for women and babies, not to improve the scientific base of the profession. It was felt that the image of research in midwifery contributed to this perceived separation of nurturing and science among some midwives but that, in fact, the two were closely related.

'The wanting to make life better for women is the primary motivation for a lot of the very best midwifery research in the country … I find it fascinating when people take the view that evidence is somehow divorced from nurturing, because actually if you look at some of the best studies and the most influential studies, they have changed practice, are written out of anger and the wish to change things on the part of the researcher.'

It was also felt that the underestimation of the 'artistic' side of practice was also reflected in published research in midwifery journals which emphasized a quantitative objective methodology. Such research was felt to be particularly difficult to interpret and apply to practice.

'Some of the research some midwives carry out tends to be more along the lines of medical type models … more quantitative type research, whereas a lot of the things we do are very interpersonal, it's very one-to-one … It's those things that we need to capture, it's those things that we need to have down on paper.'

'It's all right reading the research, but then you've got to decide if you can implement it. Is it transferable? If this piece of research has been done in some hospital in London with every facility known to man and you're in a little cottage hospital in the north of Scotland, is it going to apply?'

The group had some suggestions as to how research articles could be more accessible and appealing to practitioners, without losing their scientific quality.

'I've seen the odd article where … at the beginning they have a little case history. So, you think, oh yes I've seen this happen in practice. It makes you want to go on and read the rest of it and find out what the solutions have been.'

'Practitioners, who maybe don't feel very valued, are, perhaps, the ones who come up with some issues that they think do need looking at. They might think, "oh that's a problem" but they may not think, "oh it needs researching". It's the word research that puts a whole new connotation on things.'

CONCLUSION

Balancing the 'art and science' components of the role of the midwife is challenging. Perhaps this issue is particularly acute in midwifery because of the long tradition of working with individual women and cultivating that special relationship with them and their babies. The desire to develop generalizable research findings from studies of midwifery care which can be implemented in clinical practice is based on the same objectives – continuing to improve the care provided to women and babies.

From some of the comments made in the group, there is a perception that some fragmentation is developing in the profession, between educators, researchers and clinical midwives. This needs urgent attention, as it is by collaboration and building on shared objectives that the profession can continue to develop. There are challenges for midwives in clinical, education, managerial and research roles.

One of the many challenges lies in developing the skills to integrate the two components of art and science within everyday practice, and to ensure that research in midwifery is guided by a focus on practice. Making research more accessible to practitioners is an important priority, at the same time, continuing to develop mechanisms which enable midwives to develop skills in research appraisal and which support them to change practice and share information in a non-threatening way.

It is clear from the discussion with students and midwives, that midwifery is changing. At the start of the discussion we conducted a brain storming exercise and asked participants to name aspects of practice which they felt were based on evidence, and those they felt were not. Two lengthy lists soon emerged. Ten, even 5 years ago, would a mixed group of midwives have achieved this? Huge changes have occurred over recent years in practice, education, research and service organization. Midwives are changing, and the way they provide care and use research evidence in their practice is also changing. These are exciting, and at the same time challenging times.

'Things are changing and, in the future, there will be more people coming through who have done the courses we have and got that way of thinking. Obviously, there are qualified midwives who share the same view – it is definitely the minority who aren't so willing to change. But I think it will change naturally or progress because we will have the same philosophy and, hopefully, people will be more supportive.'

Student midwife

Acknowledgements

This valuable chapter would not have been possible without the contribution of the group members. We would like to thank midwives Val McCulloch, Fiona Meddings and Anne-Marie Keeley, and students Jane Harman, Mairaed Faughan and Sylvia Rainbow for being such informative and enthusiastic participants.

12

Developing research and evidence-based practice in midwifery – the next 20 years

Mary Renfrew and Sue Proctor

KEY ISSUES

- Research matters to practice
- Research is never comfortable
- The changing context of practice and research

- Continuing problems
- New developments and challenges
- Towards a framework for evidence-based practice.

INTRODUCTION

The chapters in this book outline the developments of research and evidence-based practice in midwifery in the UK in the past 20 years, and the strengths and challenges we face. They have some clear messages for us as we plan for the next 20 years.

RESEARCH MATTERS TO PRACTICE

Research matters to practice; midwives recognize this and are committed to using evidence-based practice (Chapters 1, 4, 8, 9, 11). There is a recognition that if we wish to offer all women, their babies and their families sensitive, skilled care which meets their needs and avoids harm, we must use and extend our knowledge about their needs, and about appropriate practices which will help to make childbearing safe and fulfilling (Chapter 7).

It is not easy to use research in practice, however (Chapters 8, 11). Skilled midwives with many years of experience already make difficult judgements based on their knowledge; adding research evidence to this makes it potentially more complicated. Midwives need support to learn how to do this, especially if they have been in practice for many years and have not had training in critical appraisal skills. A fundamental skill in midwifery is being able to blend both art and science to offer the best care. Being able to integrate knowledge derived from research with the skills of communication, judgement, decision-making and hands-on care is the basis of excellent practice (Chapter 8).

RESEARCH IS NEVER COMFORTABLE

Research is never a comfortable option (Chapters 1, 2, 4, 8, 11, probably others too!). It is challenging; it demands change, and it often does not tell you what you would like it to.

If you are a researcher, studies you carry out may come up with results you did not anticipate and you may have difficulty explaining your findings. You may even have to stand up in public and tell others about a study which you know they will not like. They may criticize you and your findings.

If you are a manager, research may indicate that you should organize your services differently. You are already stressed and do not have enough resources to run the existing service. So, research can add to the pressure you feel.

If you are a practitioner, research results may suggest that you change your practice. You may not like, or feel skilled in, the new methods. Research may suggest that what you have been doing for years is not best practice. It may even challenge your strongly-held beliefs, as was the case with the third stage trials (Chapter 2).

If you are an educator, newly published research means that you have to continue to update your teaching sessions, and you can never be completely sure that you are up to date.

If you are a student, you can't rely on what you were told remaining constant, as new research may throw new light on a topic, or suggest a practice different from the one you were taught.

If we are to offer women and babies the best possible care, we will have to adapt to the challenge of keeping up to date with research, even if we do not always like what we find. Curiosity, humility, open mindedness, a willingness to admit that you made mistakes, and a sense of humour are essential prerequisites to using, or carrying out research.

THE CHANGING CONTEXT OF PRACTICE AND RESEARCH

The context of practice and education in midwifery has changed greatly in the past 20 years (Chapters 1, 5, 7, 8, 9, 10). Positive developments include the increasing contribution of women's views to developments in practice, the availability of evidence to inform practice, and the move of midwifery education into universities. At the same time, however, midwives have been working in a health service which has become used to a chronic shortage of resources, has been reorganized several times, where education and practice have become distanced, and in which the language and concept of cost-effectiveness has become embedded in everyday thinking.

The context of research has changed almost beyond recognition

(Chapters 2, 3, 7, 11). In 1978, there was almost no research in midwifery, no midwives with research degrees, and virtually no role models of midwives involved in research. In 1998, the Midwifery Research Database (MIRIAD) had information about nearly 500 studies in the field. Midwives have PhDs and MPhil degrees. Midwives have gained funding from mainstream funding bodies, including the MRC and the NHS R&D programme, and midwives doing research can now work in a multi-disciplinary, health services research context which did not exist 20 years ago. There are academic departments of midwifery, midwife researchers, midwifery lecturers who do research, midwives working in, and leading, multi-disciplinary research groups, midwives working in clinical effectiveness posts and practice development and lecturer practitioners posts. Midwives are involved in co-ordinating national audit projects, and there are professors of midwifery. There is an annual national conference with peer-reviewed papers, acting as a scientific forum, and there will be an international version of this conference in 2001.

CONTINUING PROBLEMS

We need to be realistic, however, about our stage of development in research, and our potential to develop further (Chapters 1, 2, 8, 11). Although we have moved far in the past 20 years, it is not far or fast enough for research to underpin all of our practice, or for us to feel secure that research will continue to grow and thrive. We still find that research is patchy and of inconsistent quality. There are few trained and experienced midwife researchers, there are large numbers of midwives who have little, if any, opportunity to develop critical appraisal skills, and there is a perceived gap between research and practice.

We have a long way to go before we can live up to the challenge of the Research Assessment Exercise and be able to demonstrate consistent quality at a national and international standard in our research, or offer a high quality environment for midwives who wish to train in research. Clear thinking and planning around the best ways to link research and practice is still needed to guide the provision of the best of evidence-based practice for women and their families. There is still a tendency to think of research, practice, education and management as disconnected activities, in spite of the obvious and fundamental links between them. We still have much to debate, and to test out, before we can effectively blend the art and science of midwifery (Chapter 11).

NEW DEVELOPMENTS AND CHALLENGES

Changes in midwifery, the wider health context and society in general are likely to result in a context which will, in coming years, be more supportive of research in midwifery.

- Midwives with degrees are likely to have a different perspective on the use of knowledge in practice (Chapter 11), feel more comfortable trying new things and continuing to seek new knowledge throughout their careers. These will not only be the newly-qualified practitioners, but also the many experienced midwives who choose to continue their education.
- Women who feel able to voice their views, backed up by information about research and about care (Chapter 5), will challenge midwives to improve practice and will also support them in making changes where these are needed.
- National developments in research, including the recognition of the need to develop research capacity in non-medical health professions (Pearson 1998), the ongoing development of the NHS R&D programme (including the establishment of the Service Delivery and Organization programme), and support for research in primary care (NHS Executive 1997) all offer new opportunities for research and researchers in midwifery.
- National developments in the context of practice, including the changing and more autonomous role of midwives and multi-disciplinary developments such as the National Institute for Clinical Effectiveness (NICE), National Service Frameworks, clinical governance and audit, offer a more supportive environment for midwives to ask and answer their own questions about practice.
- New developments in information technology will make information easier to find, and more accessible.
- Developments in primary care will radically change the organization and structure of the health services (Department of Health 1997). It will result in shifting alliances – more contact with GPs, for example, perhaps less with obstetricians, and opportunities for change.

Making best use of these challenges and addressing the problems we have described, needs a proactive, strategic approach. We outline here a framework for planning the development of evidence-based practice in midwifery.

TOWARDS A FRAMEWORK FOR DEVELOPING EVIDENCE-BASED PRACTICE

Excellence in practice is underpinned by knowledge derived from research, supported by good and ongoing education and skilled change management. All those concerned with standards of practice, therefore, must be aware of the fundamental contribution of research and education to practice and the key role of management. This will include the professional and statutory bodies, trusts, and consumer groups. Similarly, those involved in planning for education, including education consortia and universities, need to understand the context of practice and the need to develop research capacity. Those involved in planning and conducting research need to be aware of clinical practice issues to help make decisions about priorities, for example, and to plan for education to support high quality training in research. Managers will find they need to understand and use knowledge derived from research and to ensure good continuing education for their staff, so that practice can be as good as possible. Excellent midwifery comprises a balance between these four parts – without the balance, each of the other areas will suffer.

Of course, many individuals work across these areas. Lecturers can work in education, practice and research. Practice development midwives can work in practice, management and research. Researchers can work in practice and education. Managers need good links in all four areas. The structure of the organization in which midwives work and the structure of the profession itself, needs to reflect and support the links between these areas.

Some of the following examples of developments might support this integrated planning and could be built into a framework at local or national levels:

1. At Trust and Primary Care Group level, both in hospital and the community, we need a strategy for finding and using information about practice and about research. This will include local information derived from audit, as well as published information about research results. Links will be needed, therefore, in the organization and delivery of audit,

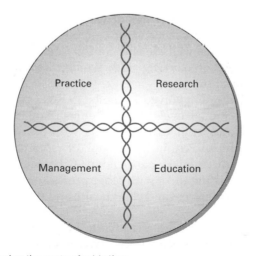

Figure 12.1   Balancing the parts of midwifery

standards development, clinical effectiveness/governance, continuing education, and research. This will include access to library facilities. A joint multi-disciplinary strategy would enable this to happen more effectively.

2. Education contracting needs to recognize that midwives should be prepared to a level where they can offer evidence-based care. This will involve ensuring that they can be taught in environments where research is valued and skills of critical appraisal are fundamental. In turn, this will have implications for the way in which resources are spent. High quality education requires that students are taught by lecturers who are active in research. They will therefore need time, resources and support to do that well.

3. Bridging the gap between research and education is one challenge – bridging the gap between both and clinical practice is another. As education has moved into universities, the experience in some places is that practice has become even more disconnected from education and research. This is not inevitable; we can address it if we face the problem and work to create and develop links. Lecturers who are active in research and practice, in practice and education, can help to bridge the gap. Midwives who understand and use research evidence in practice can support students who have a theoretical knowledge to use that in practice. Researchers who understand the up-to-date evidence can work with practitioners to develop standards of practice and with educators to inform their teaching.

4. Statutory bodies need to ensure that skills to underpin evidence-based practice are part of pre- and post-registration education. This will require thinking through the role and responsibilities of lecturers, ways of supporting them to become research-active and acknowledging the key contribution that research has to make to education, practice and management.

5. We will need to develop ways of working closely with women to make decisions about practice and also about research priorities. The mechanisms of doing this well are still not fully developed, but midwives have a strong history of working with women and this is an obvious extension of that tradition.

6. If midwives became involved in the NHS R&D programme, at local trust, regional and national levels, it would enhance our ability to influence research priorities, and to link those closely with questions arising from practice. Increasingly, success in submission of research bids is linked to collaborative, multi-disciplinary partnerships (Chapter 3). Midwives need to further develop existing links with other professions and organizations who are interested in maternal and child health and the health care services offered to them.

7. Universities and trusts are already closely connected in relation to education and research in medicine. Developing the same model for research in midwifery would enhance our ability to link academic research

and education with clinical practice. Developing a joint R&D strategy between trusts and universities, for example, would support this. Developing academic/clinical departments of midwifery would also enhance this.

8. We need to increase the numbers of midwives involved in generating knowledge, so that knowledge is appropriate to the needs of midwives, women and babies. This will require investment in research training and a career structure which enables midwives to develop in research, as well as stay within a clinical context.

9. Stable, high quality research programmes are needed to address the range of important questions about practice, dissemination and implementation. It is only by developing such programmes that substantial funding will be gained from funding agencies for programmes of work, for individual studies or for studentships. Most funding agencies like to see a track record of successful research. In addition to enhancing the quality of research, they would also offer an environment to train researchers and where those involved in practice and education could learn about research.

10. Huge variations exist in the care given to women and babies in different parts of the world. The ease with which care givers get access to evidence-based information is also incredibly variable. Midwives have an important role in working with obstetric, paediatric and public health colleagues towards developing effective links with professionals worldwide who care for women and babies. Working collaboratively and learning together can help develop practices which are both safe and effective for childbearing women and their families.

CONCLUSION

To improve the care of women and their families, to develop the midwifery profession and the use of evidence-based practice, developments in practice, research, education and management need to be more closely integrated. This needs to happen at the level of the individual and in local, regional and national organizations, so that there is a shared agenda and a sense of purpose and direction to make the care of mothers, babies and their families as good as it can be.

REFERENCES

Department of Health *The New NHS – Modern, Dependable* White Paper for England London: HMSO; 1997
NHS Executive *R&D in Primary Care – National Working Group Report* Department of Health London: HMSO; 1997
Pearson M *Developing Human resources for Health Related R&D: Next Steps* Report of the R&D workforce capacity development group London: Department of Health; 1998

Core skills for research

Some midwives may find their questions about practice cannot be answered sufficiently by reviewing existing knowledge. In such cases, it may be appropriate to conduct a study which can help provide an answer. This section does not attempt to provide a comprehensive research methods guide, as many other excellent resources exist which meet this objective. In five relatively short chapters, some of the core skills required for conducting a research study are discussed by experts in the field. In each case, there are examples and tips for the reader which may help them improve and refine their projects. These include designing a research proposal and applying to a research ethics committee. Some methodological principles are also presented. Research approaches which are popular in midwifery research are examined, such as designing a questionnaire, conducting an interview and conducting observational research. Guides for further reading are also included in each of these brief chapters.

13

Designing a research proposal

Ann Wraight

KEY ISSUES

- First, determine whether there is a definite need to do the research
- Follow the steps of the research process
- The proposal must convince the reader that the research is important

- Allow 6–12 months to design the proposal, secure approval and funding
- A hastily prepared document has a high chance of failure.

INTRODUCTION

A research project often begins with an idea – a flash of inspiration or just a slow dawning that some aspect of the care being provided needs to be changed or improved. However, before rushing off to collect data and change practice, we need to consider the potential implications of the whole job: the time, the cost, the expertise and the participants. Most of all, we need to assess whether there is a definite need to do this research in the first place and who, if anyone, will benefit. Writing the whole process down focuses the mind, clears up any confusion or doubts and produces a research proposal.

'A research proposal is a detailed statement of what you intend to do, why you intend to do it and how you intend to go about it. It indicates both to you and anyone involved with your research both your ability to carry through the project and whether the design and methods you have selected are appropriate to the problem you have selected.'

(Burnard & Morrison 1994)

The proposal has three main functions:

1. To provide the managers, supervisors or other interested parties with a written plan of the project for their consideration.
2. To submit an application to the Local Research Ethics Committee(s) for approval.
3. To submit an application to an appropriate body in order to secure funding.

Although the writing of a proposal is not simple, the completed document is useful to the researcher, both as a plan to consult throughout the whole project and as a framework for the final written report.

Some funding agencies produce their own guidelines for the submission of a research proposal but, in general, there are no set rules for the presentation or layout. The aim in the first instance is to persuade the reader to read the proposal. Therefore, it needs to be legible, attractive and written in a clear and logical sequence. Sufficient information needs to be given to allow the reader to appreciate the need and potential benefits of the proposed research without overburdening with too much unnecessary detail. The use of headings and sub-headings gives the reader an opportunity to draw breath, while diagrams and flow charts can lighten the document and clarify the plan, when used appropriately. Following the steps outlined in Box 13.1 is a simple way to prepare a proposal and helps to ensure that nothing is omitted. Once the proposal has been prepared, then the whole document or selected parts of it can be made available to the various committees, bodies, institutions and individuals as required.

Box 13.1   Proposal checklist

- Title of the proposed project
- Overview
- Background
  - The research question or hypothesis
  - Aims and objectives
  - Review of the relevant literature
- Plan of investigations
  - Research methods
  - Study population and sampling
  - Time scale
  - Ethical considerations
  - Data analysis
  - Dissemination of results
- Resources
  - Personnel
  - Budget
- Appendices

THE PROPOSAL

Title

The title of the project should be brief but explicit to provide the reader with a simple description of the proposed study. Once submitted, the project will be known by this title and it should, therefore, be short. However, some studies may be examining an issue already researched, so it is important to differentiate this project from others previously published. For example, the topic of pain in labour has been studied many times over the years, but from different perspectives and with different aims. The title of a project may need a subtitle in order to keep the main title short and yet provide enough detail to describe this specific work. For example, the National Birthday Trust study on pain in labour was titled:

(Title)   *Pain and its Relief in Childbirth*:
(subtitle) *The results of a national survey conducted by the National Birthday Trust*

(Chamberlain, Wraight & Steer 1993)

Overview

The overview of the project should be short but informative. An approximate length is 200–250 words. This is an important section of the proposal since it may be the only part read by some people, while others will read the whole document. It therefore warrants careful thought and consideration. For example, the research proposal for a project examining the issues involved in adopting a different model of care, midwifery-led care as opposed to consultant-led care, would include the following in the overview:

- The reasons for wishing to conduct the research, such as the need to demonstrate the implications to midwifery staff of the proposed changes.
- A brief description of how it will be done, e.g. a survey of all midwives providing care in hospital and community over a 6 month period.
- The perceived benefits, e.g. advantages and disadvantages of the proposed new style of care.

It is often easier to write this part of the proposal last, when the plan of the whole project has been formulated and every detail is clear in the mind of the researcher.

Background

The research question or hypothesis

A discussion of the need for and benefits of the proposed project must be presented, so that the reader becomes convinced that the study is an important one which is worth supporting. The research question needs to be stated clearly, so that no one is left in any doubt about the intention of the project or how it will be conducted. If the project is to be based on an assumption or hypothesis, then this should be presented here. The following is an example of an hypothesis: *Women who are cared for in labour by a known midwife will use less pharmacological pain relief.*

Aims and objectives

The aims and objectives of the project need to be listed in order to provide a clear statement of what will be achieved. The aim is the goal, while the objectives are more specific activities to be carried out during the process of achieving the aim. The following is an example of an aim and an objective from a study on the implications to midwives of team midwifery:

Aim: *The aim is to provide the Royal College of Midwives with a better understanding of the issues surrounding team midwifery and other ways in which midwifery has been organized to provide greater continuity of care.*

Objective 1:   *To identify processes involved in the introduction of team midwifery, including an examination of the appropriateness of the current grading system.*

(Stock & Wraight 1993)

Review of the literature

Before progressing too far through the project plan, the relevant literature needs to be reviewed to demonstrate knowledge of current research (see Chapter 6). Here, one should describe how and why previous research has been done, and demonstrate whether or not relevant evidence is available. There are three main reasons for searching the literature:

1. To gain more knowledge of the subject to be researched, or of a specific aspect, or just the clarification of a term, e.g. in the above hypothesis, what is meant by the word 'known' in this context?
2. To determine what research has been carried out already on the same or similar topics, so that unnecessary duplication does not occur, and lessons can be learned from the advice and experience of others.
3. To identify the appropriate methods of data collection by discussing the various options and justifying the reasons for the methods of choice.

Plan of investigations

Research methods

A general description of the research design and methods to be used for data collection must be provided. For example, if it is planned to use a questionnaire, the reasons for choosing this method as opposed to any other, such as interviews, should be outlined. It is important to note whether the questionnaire has been used before or whether it is newly constructed. If it has not been tried and tested in another study, then a discussion on the intention of checking for validity and reliability would give strength to the proposal at this stage.

Study population and sampling

A description of the proposed study population needs to be included – who will be invited to participate, how many and in what locality? Details ot the sampling technique and exclusion criteria must be given, unless a whole population over a period of time, such as all women who attend the antenatal clinic in the first week of June, is to be chosen. Even then, justification of your choice of that specific week is required. Evidence of your communication with the appropriate authority for possible access to the subjects should also be included.

Time scale

A start and completion date for the planned research is essential, but if funding has not been gained, finalizing these dates is difficult. A timetable to indicate the full duration and occurrence of the various stages is very helpful to the sponsor, as well as to the grant holder and the researcher. It requires care to produce this plan since underestimation may jeopardize the whole project. Generally, more time is needed at the planning stages than is usually allocated: allow for communication, ethics approval and the design and testing of the data collection tools.

Some activities end before the next one starts, for example questionnaire design must be completed before the questionnaires can be printed and despatched. Many activities, however, overlap, and the researcher's time allocation will vary according to the needs of the different stages of the project. Consideration of all the personnel involved, their other commitments and holiday periods should be addressed in addition to size of sample, time span for recruitment and pilot studies. Always allow longer for each stage than is first thought to be necessary. Table 13.1 is an example of a timetable which could apply to a 2 year study involving a postal questionnaire survey.

Ethical considerations

As the research plan progresses, consideration needs to be given to ethical

Table 13.1 Study timetable

	Year 1	Year 2
Communication with all involved	....	....
Preparation of questionnaires	....	
Pilot study	....	
Despatch of questionnaires:		
main sample	....	
follow-up sample	....	...
Coding of questionnaires	....	.....
Data entering	....	....
Data analysis and editing		....
Writing report		....
Feedback of local results		...

issues which will or may arise in the course of the project (see Chapter 4). A discussion on how these will be handled should be included. For example, informed consent from the research participants will need to be obtained before any data can be collected. An information sheet, consent form and a plan of how the subjects will be invited to participate all need to be documented within the proposal (see Chapter 14). If a vulnerable group, for example, neonates are to be involved, then specific details should be given regarding the informed consent of the parents. It must be demonstrated that the study includes safeguards to ensure confidentiality, that no harm will be caused to the participants and that they have been assured they have the right to withdraw from the study at any time without causing an interference to their care.

Data analysis

For quantitative studies, the help of a statistician should be enlisted early on in the research design so that both the researcher and the reader feel confident that the chosen method has been examined fully and is appropriate to meet the aims and objectives. The reader will be considering at this point whether the research question is answerable. At this stage, a short description of the strategy plan, the rationale for the planned sample size and the outcome measures to be assessed should be sufficient explanation. It is helpful to give an indication of the methods of data analysis to be used. If a computer is to be used for the storage and analysis of the data, then the implications of the Data Protection Act must be discussed, such as anonymity, password protection and long-term data access.

Dissemination of results

An important part of a research study is the dissemination of the results so that others can benefit from the knowledge gained. A discussion of how this will be done should be included. Reporting the findings of the study to the participants and others who were involved in the project is essential, so that they feel rewarded for their work and also so that they can reflect on whether changes need to be implemented. This practice also improves the reputation of the researcher. The results also need to be published on a larger scale in appropriate professional journals, national newspapers or magazines, and presented at conferences and study days.

Resources

Personnel

Reference needs to be made to everyone who will be involved in the research study. This will include members of the project team if the researcher is undertaking the study jointly with colleagues or other researchers; members of an advisory team or steering committee if one has been set up; experts in research design, statistics, computer programming, economics or any other aspect relevant to the project.

Budget

If funds are being sought, a list of estimates for the various items of expenditure will be required. This is as difficult to produce as the timetable since a fine line must be drawn between overestimating the cost, which may decrease the chance of securing financial support, and underestimating the cost, which may provide insufficient funds. Competition for funds for research projects is keen and it will be noted if application for unreasonable items is made. For example, justification for the purchase of such expensive items of equipment as a computer and printer would need to be argued. If the project is long term – 3 years or more – then it is always wise to add on 10–15% to allow for inflation. The cost of advertisements for new posts tends to be underestimated. An advertisement in a national newspaper can cost in the region of £1000. Universities and some other institutions require researchers to add overhead costs of more than 40% to all grants submitted to the Research Councils and the NHS Research and Development programme. This is used to support central university costs, for example, accommodation and staffing. Charities do not pay this overhead. The total costs can be divided into capital costs, such as equipment, and recurring costs, such as postage and travel. Table 13.2 is an example of a budget showing categories which are applicable to many midwifery and nursing projects.

Table 13.2 Proposed study budget

Item	Expenditure (£)	
	Year 1	Year 2
Research midwife: interviews; 3 months	2500	
Secretarial support	1500	1000
Travel		250
Printing/photocopying	300	100
Postage	50	50
Office costs	250	250
Honorarium for statistician	500	500
Data preparation		1000
Stationery	200	100
Telephone	100	50
15% overheads to cover administration, library etc.		1305
Sub total	5400	4605
Total		10 005

Appendices

The following may be appended to the proposal:

- a sample of the data collection form, e.g. a questionnaire or structured interview form
- a sample of the information sheet and consent form to be given to the participants
- a curriculum vitae of each member of the project team
- a glossary of medical and technical terms used in the proposal
- references referred to in the proposal.

SUMMARY OF MAIN POINTS IN DESIGNING A RESEARCH PROPOSAL

A hastily prepared document which does not provide adequate information about the proposed project from start to finish has a high chance of failure. The time required to write a proposal and to secure approval and funding is lengthy (it can take between 6 and 12 months). This must be taken into consideration at the very beginning of the planning stage. It is wise to seek the advice and constructive criticism of experienced researchers during the design process of the proposal and before submitting it to the relevant funding bodies. Whether you are a novice or an expert in the field of research, other researchers will not only give advice about the contents or layout of the proposal but will also provide encouragement if patience and resilience have reached a low ebb.

Producing a proposal is a time-consuming but essential task. Whether its aim is to secure funds, ethics approval or access to potential research participants, it needs to attract the readers and convince them that this is a study worthy of their support.

FURTHER READING

Haggard MP 'Writing Research Proposals' *Current Obstetrics and Gynaecology* 1996; **6(2):** 119–121
This paper provides some useful practical tips for anyone preparing a research proposal. Professor Haggard gives advice on aspects which need to be considered fully before the application is made, otherwise it will result in failure. For example, the justification for public or charity money to be invested in the project needs to be clearly identified:

1. Why the research question is important?
2. What is the long term potential for health gain?
3. Does a professional channel exist which can make use of the results?

National Board for Nursing, Midwifery and Health Visiting for Scotland *Guidelines on Writing a Research Proposal* Edinburgh: NBS; 1995
This booklet is targeted at first time researchers although it can also be of assistance to more experienced ones too. The guidelines are easy to follow and apply. As well as including a list of references and bibliography, it also illustrates each section with quotes from nurse

researchers. A helpful example of how the total funding needs to be itemized to show categories of expenditure is included.

Sleep J *Writing a Research Proposal and Applying for Funding* London: RCM; 1989
This short booklet is easily read and has the benefit of providing guidelines, not just on the writing of the proposal, but also the process of applying for funding. Although it provides a brief overview, it covers all the main points and includes a list of useful addresses and references.

REFERENCES

Burnard P, Morrison P *Nursing Research in Action* Second edition London: Macmillan; 1994
Chamberlain G, Wraight A, Steer P *Pain and its Relief in Childbirth* London: Churchill Livingstone; 1993
Stock J, Wraight A *Developing Continuity of Care in Maternity Services* London: Institute of Manpower Studies; 1993

14

Applying to a Local Research Ethics Committee

Ray Field

KEY ISSUES

- The functions of Local Research Ethics Committees and Multi-Centre Research Ethics Committees.
- The different decisions available to the LREC regarding submitted research proposals.
- The typical questions an LREC might ask to decide on the ethical validity of a research proposal.

- What needs to be considered by the researcher to ensure they obtain informed consent.
- An example of a 'Participant Information Sheet'.
- The practical steps of how to apply to a research ethics committee and what to include in a proposal.

INTRODUCTION

In Chapter 4 Hazel McHaffie outlined the reasons for an ethical approach to research and the principles that should be considered when designing and carrying out research. This chapter concentrates on the practicalities of applying to a Local Research Ethics Committee (LREC). What are they? Who are they? What types of research need their approval? What will they be looking for? How should you prepare an application form that will be approved?

LOCAL RESEARCH ETHICS COMMITTEES

Background

In the United Kingdom, since 1967, there have been LRECs. These committees are accountable ultimately to the Secretary of State. Their membership includes medical, nursing and midwifery professionals, a general practitioner, a legal professional and at least two lay members. The members are appointed not as representatives of their own profession or interest group, but in their own right, as individuals with relevant experience to make informed judgment of the research protocols. Their function is to satisfy themselves about the ethics of all research proposals which are health related, and they must be consulted about any research involving:

1. Human participants including NHS patients (i.e. participants recruited by virtue of past or present treatment by the NHS), fetal material, in vitro fertilization and the recently dead. (This includes those treated under contract with private sector providers.)
2. Access to records and names of past and present NHS patients.
3. The use of, or potential access to, NHS premises or facilities.

Research in midwifery is likely to include one or more of these categories, but some are less relevant to the midwife researcher. The location of the participants usually determines if the researcher needs to consult the LREC. An independent midwife working outside the NHS employment framework may need approval of the LREC if their research involves NHS patients. The approval of the LREC should be seen as a helpful independent safeguard, rather than an unnecessary hurdle to be overcome. LRECs interpret differently the requirement for the above three categories of research to be approved; for example, some committees require approval for research projects involving nurses, midwives and colleagues as participants. This is to ensure that staff groups are not being asked to participate in research which has not made adequate arrangements for their consent to participate, anonymity, and confidentiality.

Researchers can believe, or be incorrectly advised by their supervisor, that if their research does not involve patients, then there is no need to apply for ethical approval to the LREC. This is not always the case and each LREC will have its own policy. Colleagues, nurses and midwives are entitled to the same protection from harm and reassurance that their rights of informed consent, confidentiality and anonymity are considered.

Audit

A further issue frequently raised with LRECs is whether audit needs their approval. LRECs do not approve clinical audit, as it is regarded as a review of normal clinical practice and institutional systems, usually against a given or accepted standard. Research, on the other hand, has been described as the systematic collection of data for the purpose of prediction or explanation. The difference between audit and research is not always clear and the reader is advised, if in doubt, to seek the opinion of their local LREC (the subject of audit is discussed in Chapter 9). A report from the Royal College of Physicians (1996) has described the difference between research and audit with the adage 'research is finding out what you ought to be doing; audit is seeing whether you are doing what you ought to be doing.'

MULTI-CENTRE RESEARCH ETHICS COMMITTEES

Multi-centre Research Ethics Committees (MRECs) are in place in each of the eight English NHS Regions, with similar arrangements in place for Scotland, Wales and Northern Ireland (Department of Health 1997). The Regional Research & Development Directorate has the responsibility for overseeing the function of the MREC. There are 15 to 18 members on each MREC drawn from the general public, pharmacy, medicine in hospital and community, nursing, midwifery, and from professions allied to health and social sciences. Any research carried out within *five* or more local LRECs' geographical boundaries should be submitted to the MREC for the region where the principal researcher is located. The MREC reviews the research for and on behalf of all the other local LRECs, who receive a summary of the outcome and can accept or reject the protocol for local reasons, but are not allowed to change the substance of the protocol.

What do LRECs do?

The LREC acts on behalf of the Health Authority in England, or equivalent authority in Scotland, Wales and Northern Ireland. The committee reviews research proposals being undertaken in the Trusts and community services which operate under its jurisdiction. The committee decides if a research proposal can commence in the Health Authority area it covers. The decisions available to the committee are:

1. approve
2. approve subject to amendment
3. request amendment prior to approval
4. reject.

It is important to note that an LREC only approves research projects for their *ethical acceptability*. Access to the hospital or community services to carry out the research is a local management decision, and must be negotiated separately with those who manage the proposed research site, and with clinicians responsible for patients who may be invited to participate in a study.

What do LRECs look for?

The Department of Health in its Briefing Pack for LRECs (Department of Health 1997) offers three different ways of approaching ethical issues in research proposals. The Committee will have detailed questions to ask under each heading, which include:

1. Validity of the research
2. Welfare of research participants
3. Dignity of the research participants.

Validity of the research

What question is the research project addressing?
Have the researchers clearly described the exact question to which they are seeking an answer, or is the proposal attempting to gather information on too wide a range of issues?
How important is the research question?
Is the question being asked important? If the participants are to give up their time to answer questions which may be embarrassing or intrusive, then the research question should be important enough to warrant taking up patients' or colleagues' time and effort. That the research question is interesting to the researcher, or that they need to complete a project as part of a degree or diploma course is not sufficient reason in itself to undertake the research. The committee is keen to know if the research question has already been answered by another study, and if so why is it being repeated. The committee will question any proposed benefit for the patients taking part in the research. That the results may benefit patients in the future, may not be sufficient justification for undertaking the research with the current group of participants.
Can the research answer the question being asked?
Is the research the right design to get an answer to the question being asked? Research that is poorly designed without clear endpoints and measures of outcome, can waste time and inconvenience people, which is unethical.
Is the researcher suitably qualified, supported and capable of doing the research?
The researcher should be sufficiently professionally qualified to understand the question being addressed and deal with any possible conflicts of interest. The midwife does not need to be an expert researcher to do research as this expertise can be provided by the research supervisor or colleagues. The researcher should, however, be sufficiently aware of issues relating to confidentiality and their professional code of practice, to avoid exposing the participants to unnecessary risk.
Are the facilities for the research appropriate?
The researcher should ensure that the environment where the study is being undertaken is adequate. It is unethical to ask people to speak to a researcher on an open ward, or antenatal clinic, for all to overhear. Similarly, asking people to be interviewed at home for several hours, or to complete a personal questionnaire at their workplace may not be an appropriate environment for the research.
How will progress and the findings be disseminated?
The LREC may wish to see reporting arrangements in place to ensure that the researcher updates them about the progress of the study, or advises them of any problems as they arise. This may be particularly relevant when the research topic is sensitive, for example, women's experience of stillbirth

or postnatal depression, where the research process may have a greater effect on the participants or service than was expected.

Welfare of the research participant

What will participating in the research involve?

The LREC will take account of the research procedures from the participant's point of view and will consider their welfare. Procedures to obtain for example, a blood sample, smear test, or urine sample, may be harmful, uncomfortable, or just inconvenient. The committee will be concerned if participants are being asked to stay longer at a clinic, or in hospital, or spend extra time answering questions beyond the normal length of the visit or consultation. If participants are being asked to travel to meet the researcher, or attend for extra visits, then their travelling expenses or reasonable child-care expenses may have to be paid. The researcher should consider carefully and seek expert advice regarding provision for indemnity and compensation in the event of injury due to participation in the study. Further information is available in *NHS Indemnity – Arrange ments for Clinical Negligence Claims in the NHS* (1996).

Are any risks necessary and are they acceptable?

The researcher may wish to balance some risk against the benefit of doing the research. There may be some risk inherent in the research process, for example interviewing people at home, or alone, which may put t he researcher at risk. The nature of research may add extra risk to the participants' safety or well-being, for example asking them questions which may stir up unpleasant memories of previous miscarriages, still-births, or the history of a traumatic delivery. This may result in them feeling depressed or anxious.

Dignity of the research participant

Will consent be sought?

The issue of consent is at the heart of research and as noted in *A Charter for Ethical Research in Maternity Care* (NCT 1998), when a woman is pregnant, in labour, or breastfeeding, she is consenting to take part in research for two people, herself and her child. An important consideration for the LREC is to ensure that the participant's consent is sought to take part in the study. Absence of consent may constitute an offence against the person (assault and battery) or a legal wrong (tort). The participant's consent should be voluntary and not influenced by a desire to avoid disapproval of, or to please, the researcher, particularly where they are also the midwife.

Will the consent be verbal or written?

It is good practice to provide the participant with a written information sheet well in advance of being asked for consent to participate in research.

Box 14.1 outlines some considerations in devising an information sheet, and Box 14.2 illustrates an example. Most LRECs will regard a well written information sheet and separate consent form as the gold standard. This was recommended by the International Conference on Harmonisation Guidelines for Good Clinical Practice (ICH 1997)

If colleagues, nurses or midwives are participants, they also require adequate information and a consent form. An LREC would need to be convinced to deviate from this requirement and approve verbal consent. In exceptional circumstances the LREC might regard verbal consent as acceptable, possibly on the grounds of the particular design of the study, such as the use of a short questionnaire. If used, verbal consent should be witnessed and recorded by the researcher. In addition to written information sheets, researchers could consider using videos or audio tapes to explain the research proposal to the participants. Special arrangements should be made to meet the needs of those people who have disabilities, reading difficulties, different languages or cultural backgrounds. The information sheet should be given to the participant in advance of the actual research, so that they and, if appropriate, their family can think matters over, before consenting to take part, or not.

Box 14.1 Participant information sheet

Introduction
The title should be in simple English (or other appropriate language), with the purpose of the research study explained in plain, concise terms and avoiding jargon. How and why they have been chosen to participate should be explained.

What will I have to do if I take part?
The participant should be informed about the data collection method: for example, questionnaire, interview, focus group, if it will be taped, and how long it will take. Any extra clinical procedures, visits, clinic attendances should all be explained. If they are to receive travelling expenses, this should be explained.

What are the possible risks of taking part?
Any possible risks, side effects, discomfort or emotional effects of taking part in the research, for both the participant and their family should be described.

Are there any benefits to taking part?
If there is benefit to the participant from being in the study, this should be described. That the research is part of the midwife's degree or diploma studies is not a benefit to the participant.

Do I have to take part?
The voluntary nature of the study must be clearly stated. If the participant would prefer not to take part they do not have to give a reason. That their treatment or care will not be affected should be made clear, also that they can change their mind at any time without giving a reason.

Who to contact?
One person the participant can contact to discuss the study (if they so wish) and how to do this should be described. Details of appropriate advocates, community health council members may be helpful to provide the participant with an independent view.

Box 14.2   Example of a participant information sheet

Title of project
Predicting breast feeding intentions, influencing factors and behaviour among first time mothers who initially intend to breast feed.

Explanation of the project
I would like to invite you to participate in this important research study. It aims to learn about your attitudes while you are pregnant to breast feeding, and what influences your choice during pregnancy about whether or not you intend to breast feed your baby. It also aims to learn about and understand your experiences of feeding your baby – what is important to you – and the care or advice you find helpful or unhelpful.

   This information will be invaluable in helping us to give women who want to breast feed the most useful support and information through their pregnancy, so they feel prepared. It will also inform midwives who support and advise breast feeding mothers. The information you provide in this study will help them give care that is of most use and high quality in meeting the needs of new mothers and their babies.

Involvement in the study
If you would like to take part in the study, after reading this leaflet you will be invited to complete a consent form by your midwife. She will send this to Jane Smith, the midwife researcher. You will be asked to participate in four brief (no longer than 20 minutes maximum) telephone interviews.

- Within a couple of weeks Jane will telephone you and ask you some brief questions.
- Later in your pregnancy (when you are about 36 weeks pregnant), she will phone you again, and complete an interview about your views and experiences.
- After you have had your baby and return home, another telephone interview will be arranged and conducted at a time convenient to you.
- Finally, about 6 weeks after the birth, a final 'phone interview will be arranged and conducted.

At any time, should you no longer wish to be involved in the study, you are free to opt out of any further interviews.

I would like to assure you that the information you give will be treated in the strictest confidence. The answers to the interview questions will be coded so that your responses cannot be personally identified from the database. All the information you give will *only be used by the researcher* for the purposes of the study.

   If you would like further details about this study, please feel free to contact me on 0181 123 4507, and I will be delighted to answer any queries you might have.

   I do hope you feel able to participate in this study. Please indicate on the attached consent form whether or not you would like to be involved, and hand it to your midwife.

Thank you for your time, and best wishes for a successful pregnancy and birth.

Is the person legally competent to give consent?

The researcher should ensure that the participant can understand the nature and purpose of the proposed interventions and be able to make a decision based on this information. The researcher should seek expert advice if there is any doubt as to the participant's capacity to give informed consent. Young people of 16 and above are legally entitled to consent to treatment and thus to therapeutic research. The position regarding young people under 16 is complex and children who have the capacity and understanding to take decisions about their own treatment are able to do so in relation to therapeutic research. If the child is under 16 and not competent to give consent, parents or another person with parental responsibility, may consent on behalf of a child to therapeutic research (Foster 1997). Any objection from the child would be considered to overrule parental consent to the child's participation in research.

Will confidentiality be respected?

Researchers should ensure that information obtained from participants, written or verbal, is kept confidential and that the data are secured against unauthorized access. No individual should be identifiable from published results. If the researchers have used colleagues as research participants and assured them of their anonymity, then care must be taken not to enable the reader of the research to work out their identity. For example, identifying the respondent from the descriptor 'a senior midwife in the labour ward' may be easy, if there is only one senior midwife in the labour ward.

How to apply to an LREC

Having considered who the committee members are, what they look for, and how to prepare the proposal, before commencing their study the researcher must apply to the LREC. Often, the majority of submissions are rejected because the application forms are incomplete and do not include an example of the Participant Information Sheet or Consent Form. Before applying a researcher should consider the points outlined in Box 14.3.

Box 14.3 Planning a submission to a LREC

1. Speak to the secretary or chair of the LREC to get a copy of the application form. All sections of the application form should be completed. LRECs do not normally accept proposals unless they are typed.
2. Ensure you know the dates for submission of the research proposal and meet the deadlines.
3. If you think the proposal may contain particular ethical problems, speak to the LREC's chair or include your concerns in the proposal.
4. Find out from the secretary of the LREC if they have particular requests, for example, the need for extra photocopies of the submission.
5. Prior to submission, obtain from the relevant clinical manager and consultant *permission to gain access* to the research site. Attach a copy of the permission to the application form.
6. If your research is part of a degree or diploma course ensure your research supervisor has read and signed the proposal.
7. Include a completed copy of the Participant Information Sheet and Consent Form.
8. Ensure you are aware of any indemnity arrangements for participants. Again, if unsure, speak to the secretary of the LREC before you submit the proposal, rather than when it is returned rejected.

CONCLUSION

The LREC has a duty to their Local Health Authority to ensure that research in the NHS should conform to codes of good practice to protect participants from harm, to preserve their rights and to reassure the public that this is being done. Their role is also to advise researchers and discuss with them any ethical issues in their proposed research. They are not a faceless foreboding committee, but a group of lay people and professionals who are happy to engage in a discussion with the researcher and find solutions to ethical problems. They are there to ensure that research is not done *to* people, but rather *with* them and that time has been taken to explain and engage them in the research, if they so wish. The LREC is constantly balancing benefit of research against risk and discomfort to the participant. The midwife researcher should welcome their independent review as a helpful second opinion. The public can know that the researcher is not the sole judge of whether the research proposal conforms with codes of good practice.

FURTHER READING

Foster C *Manual for Local Research Ethics Committees* Volume 1 and 2 London: The Centre of Medical Law and Ethics King's College; 1997.
The 'Manual' is the standard reference book for LREC members in that it contains the relevant guidelines issued by the Department of Health, the Royal Colleges, the ABPI, the BMA and others. It is a detailed manual and not an easy read, but a definitive reference for those seeking guidance on specific technical questions.
Local Research Ethics Committees HSG (91) 5 Department of Health London: HMSO; 1991
This is another guidance document for LREC members and interested researchers. It is commonly known as the 'The Red Book' and contains specific guidance to LREC members on the conduct and procedures of ethics committees.
Royal College of Nursing *Ethics Related to Research in Nursing* Middlesex: RCN, Scutari; 1993
This is a less technical document that discusses general issues related to research, such as consent and confidentiality and should be on the reading list of all researchers.
British Paediatric Association *Guidelines for the Ethical Conduct of Medical Research involving Children* London: Regents Park; 1992
These guidelines are issued for paediatricians conducting research with children. However, this should not deter the general reader as it deals with the specialist subject of consenting children for research and the special legal considerations required.
NHS Executive *NHS Indemnity – Arrangements for Clinical Negligence Claims in the NHS* HSG (96) 48 London: Department of Health; 1996
This is a specialist paper outlining the agreed arrangements for non-negligent harm in clinical trials sponsored by the pharmaceutical industry. It deals with compensation for research participants in the case of negligent harm. It is essential that researchers undertaking research as NHS employees clarify their legal position with regard to issues of compensation in the event of injury for those participating in research.
Royal College of Physicians *Guidelines on the Practice of Ethics Committees in Medical Research Involving Human Participants* Third edition London: RCP 1996
This is a well written guideline that covers all the main issues related to undertaking research; consent, confidentiality, legal competence, patient information. It is written with a particular quantitative bias and with the medical researcher in mind but remains a good source book for the general researcher.
Evans D, Evans M *A Decent Proposal* Chichester, West Sussex: John Wiley & Sons; 1996

This book is an excellent guide to reviewing research within an ethical framework. It is recommended for all new LREC members, and for researchers it outlines the issues that the LREC will be considering with regard to your research.

Tarling M, Crofts L *The Essential Researcher's Handbook, For Nurses and Health Care Professionals* London: Baillière Tindall; 1989

This book deals very well with the practicality of research and explains from experience the different pitfalls that can delay and frustrate along the way. It provides helpful checklists for all nurses and midwives undertaking research.

REFERENCES

Royal College of Physicians of London *Guidelines on the Practice of Ethics Committees in Medical Research Involving Human Participants* Third edition London: RCP; 1966

Department of Health *Ethics Committee Review of Multi-centre Research* HSG(97)23 London: HMSO; 1997

Foster C *Manual for Local Research Ethics Committees* Volume 2 Section II London: The Centre of Medical Law and Ethics King's College; 1997

International Conference on Harmonisation Guideline for Good Clinical Practice Maidenhead Berks: ACRPI; 1997

National Childbirth Trust *A Charter for Ethical Research in Maternity Care* London: National Childbirth Trust; 1998

NHS Indemnity – Arrangements for Clinical Negligence Claims in the NHS HSG(96)48 London: NHS Executive; 1996

15

Questionnaire design

Gillian Wright

KEY ISSUES

- Thinking through the study objectives
- Different types of questions

- Measuring attitudes
- Designing questionnaires for self-completion

INTRODUCTION

Questionnaires are not an exact science. They do not and are not intended to offer the proof claimed by scientific or medical experiment. Rather, they are about finding patterns in what people do and think. If well designed, they can give reliable insight into the way in which behaviours and attitudes are distributed in the sample being studied. The most important issue then in questionnaire design is to decide what the *objectives* are for the study. This chapter addresses the possible objectives and the implications of these for the design of the data collection tool. Questionnaires can be a part of a range of different research designs, including surveys and randomized controlled trials.

What we actually want is the answers. It is only by asking questions that we can get to the answers. More precisely, it is only by asking the right questions that we get to the answers about the issues in which we are really interested. At an even more simplistic level, we will not get the answers to questions we do not ask. We are all likely to have been in a situation when we have not given information that we know is wanted because we have been able to interpret a question in a spurious way. For example, when asking 'was that expensive?' somebody may mean they are interested in the price you paid. But you can answer 'no' or 'half price' or 'a bargain, in the sale'. We know what someone wants to know, but if they don't ask, we're not telling!

BEFORE YOU START

Being informed

Before you even begin to consider undertaking a study, you need to be informed thoroughly about the issues you want to research. You may have information from other studies, from the health centre, hospital records and administration, health authorities or the Department of Health. You will have carried out a thorough literature review (see Chapter 6). You may also have undertaken interviews to establish the issues you want to cover and the vocabulary used by the people who will be your sample for the study.

Study objectives

Be clear that you have specific, written objectives for the questionnaire, against which you can judge the tool when it is developed. These will relate to the overall research project and to the objectives of this part of the study in particular. The objectives will be driven by whether you want a *snapshot* of the current situation or a measure of the impact of the implementation of a new policy or regime (*a longitudinal study*). Some possible generic objectives may be:

- To describe the sample (e.g. age, marital status, size of family).
- To describe behaviour (what people do).
- To understand attitudes (what do people think now, what people want and what they actually get).
- To facilitate changing attitudes (e.g. discover the importance of beliefs in different aspects of care).
- To understand how attitudes have changed (such as towards alternative therapies).
- To evaluate the impact of a policy (such as team midwifery) on women's satisfaction.
- To compare two alternatives (traditional and team midwifery).

Each of these can be made specific to your own study.

Some questionnaire jargon

People involved in questionnaire design must always look to the analysis. The responses to each question will be summarized to establish how the total sample and sub-sets of it have responded to each question. Ultimately, all individuality will be removed from the responses to give summary statistics of how each question has been answered. Each questionnaire completed by a different woman will be known as a *case* and each piece of data collected by a question, as a *variable*. The alternative responses (for example 1 = yes, 2 = no), will be known as a *value*. It is *how many* and *what type* of people respond with the alternatives you present to them that is the *feature of your analysis*.

Types of question

By asking questions, you will find out what people think; what their perceptions are. The truth as you know it, or think you know it, is one thing. But, if you know the answers, why ask the questions? People will give you the answers to the questions you ask as *they* see the situation. You should accept this information and remember that it is what you want to know. You might ask people what they are, what they do, or what they think; each of these types of question has different implications.

Non-Questions (pre-coding)

You may have information about sub-groups of your sample which you can include on the form yourself and which you do not have to ask as questions. Examples of this include which consultant a woman is registered with, whether it is her first or subsequent pregnancy, which health centre she is registered with. You can put a code on the questionnaire or even use different coloured paper for some of these variables; for example for sub-groups of pregnant and postnatal women.

What are you? (descriptors)

These descriptive questions are essential for analysis, as they are your *dependent variables*. This means that you must collect the information from individuals if you want to analyse the difference in attitudes between different groups. These may include age, socio-economic group, number of children, and marital status. If one of your objectives is to determine if attitude or behaviour is dependent on these characteristics, you need to include the appropriate classification questions. They are best placed at the end of the questionnaire as they do not actually address the subject matter of the study and so can be distracting at the beginning.

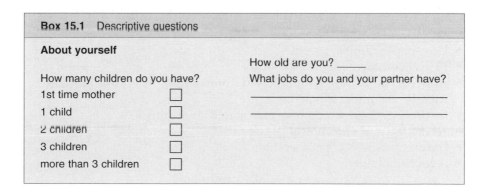

Box 15.1 Descriptive questions

About yourself

How old are you? _____

How many children do you have?   What jobs do you and your partner have?

1st time mother ☐

1 child ☐ _____

2 children ☐ _____

3 children ☐

more than 3 children ☐

Asking the age of a participant allows you to set some categories for analysis. Remember that you can always reduce the number of categories you have by combining them, but if you pre-set categories in the questionnaire (such as age groups of 16 and under, 17–21 etc) you cannot split them up later. Knowing the occupation of participants enables you to interpret their socio-economic group; you would code each participant for group using their job as an indicator of the social group variable. You have to be sure that such indicative variables are valid; for social group, you may combine income, education or other lifestyle indicators of this.

What do you do? (behavioural)

Behavioural questions are perhaps the best example to use to highlight the fact that the answers you get to any question you ask will be based on the participants' perceptions. Behaviour is, of course, a fact. You are asking people to remember behaviour and to report it accurately. With every good intention, you will get responses based on the best efforts of memories of events which have only been a small part of busy lives. Ask yourself how much you spent on groceries last month or how many beers you drank last week and you immediately see the difficulty in the self-reporting of behaviour. If behaviour can be confirmed by other sources (medical records for example), you may collect more accurate data, though you are trading off the difficulty of matching information on a respondent from two sources. It may well be as interesting to obtain the *perceptions* of behaviour from the participant. This sort of behavioural question may cover issues such as meeting the midwife, and attending antenatal groups.

What do you think? (attitudinal)

Questionnaires are often aimed at finding the views, attitudes and opinions of different groups of people. The basis for such questions may be interviews with women or service providers, or it may be that you want to know reactions to current service arrangements and processes. Some ground rules for attitude statements include:

- Use simple, familiar words.
- Keep questions as short as possible.
- Address one issue at a time. Avoid, for example, 'was your midwife friendly *and* informative?'
- Be precise; avoid words like 'reasonable' and 'sufficient'.
- Avoid medical or technical jargon.
- Ensure questions are not leading.
- Avoid ambiguity.
- Consider emotive issues especially carefully.

Measuring attitudes

Attitudes have two important features. Firstly, they have direction (*valence*): they can be positive or negative, you can agree or disagree, something can be important or unimportant. Secondly they have *strength* or *depth*, you can feel mildly or strongly about an issue. Some women feel strongly about breastfeeding (or not breastfeeding), some about natural childbirth. Understanding which women care about these issues can help to provide appropriate information and services that are well targeted. Addressing direction and depth in a questionnaire has implications for the wording of questions. What is the opposite end of a scale with 'very important' at one end? It could be 'not important' or it could be 'very unimportant'. Neither is correct. Rather, they are different scales, one measures *importance* and the other gives insight into the *direction* of the attitude as well as the *depth* of the attitude. Which one to use depends on your objectives. The important thing is to realize that asking *how* important something is different to asking *if* something is important (see Box 15.2).

Box 15.2 Scale responses
On a scale of 1–10, how important to you is:

On a scale of 1–10, how important to you is:

the option of natural childbirth   1   2   3   4   5   6   7   8   9   10

Please circle the response to the following statements that most closely defines your own opinion.

	Strongly agree	Slightly agree	No opinion	Slightly disagree	Strongly disagree
Natural childbirth is important to me	1	2	3	4	5

	Slightly agree				Strongly agree
Natural childbirth is important to me	1	2	3	4	5

Ranking

Questionnaires can include questions which ask participants to prioritize issues. These ranking questions are useful if you want to force people to make choices. These are, however, relatively difficult questions to answer and do have some limitations in analysis. The mental process of ranking means considering a number of items at once and identifying which is the *most* important. The participant must then consider the lesser list and identify the next most important and so on. Typically, in answering such questions, the most and least important issues are relatively easy for the participant to identify. The middle alternatives may not be so clear and may be ranked almost arbitrarily. If you do want to use a ranking,

Box 15.3 Attitude statements

How important are the following aspects of maternity care to you?

Please circle the response that most closely defines your own opinion.

	very important	important	no opinion	un-important	very un-important
Regular contact with midwife	1	2	3	4	5
Choice of natural childbirth	1	2	3	4	5
Information on childcare	1	2	3	4	5
Choice of hospitals	1	2	3	4	5
Information on pain control	1	2	3	4	5

How important are the following aspects of maternity care to you?

Please rank them in order 1–5, where 1 is the most important.

	Rank
Regular contact with midwife	____
Choice of natural childbirth	____
Information on childcare	____
Choice of hospitals	____
Information on pain control	____

make sure that the items are easy to understand, are comparable and that the instructions are very clear (see Box 15.3).

A major problem with ranking is that you do not know the relative distance between the rankings for each participant. It could be that for some people, only one issue is really important and so for them, number two is relatively unimportant. Conversely for others, it could be that all of the items are important and it is difficult to put them in order. Also, be quite sure how you are going to present the results. An alternative to ranking, is to present each item as an attitude statement and ask if each is important. This has the advantages of being a more sensitive measure, allowing the respondent to consider one issue at a time, to tell you that all (or none) of the items are important – it gives you a larger amount of information whilst being easier for the participant to answer.

CONDUCTING THE STUDY

The basic choice is between self-completion and interviewer involvement, either personally or by telephone. The main research implications (apart from the considerations of cost and sample size) are two fold. Firstly, that with self completion, the researcher cannot clarify anything about the instructions for completion or the questions themselves. On the other hand, the personality or presence of the interviewer cannot influence the responses in any way. Secondly, the presentation of the questionnaire is much more important when the form is self-completed and can be designed to help the respondent to reply more easily to the questions.

Box 15.4 Example of introductory statement

Breast or Bottle, what do you think?

This questionnaire is to help us improve the way you get information about breast feeding. We want to know your own views, whether you have had children or are about to have your first baby. Please tell us exactly what you think. It is only by knowing what people like you think that we can improve our service. All forms returned will be entered into a draw for a £50 Mothercare (Oddbins etc) voucher to say thanks for your help.

Design for self-completion

- Splitting the form into sections gives the impression of a number of smaller tasks, rather than giving the participant a larger task of working through a long list of questions. This follows the principle that people generally split any task into the smallest components and address a number of small tasks rather than large, complex tasks.
- Use boxes and headings to split the questionnaire. Sections headed *What has been your experience of pregnancy?*, *What is important to you about your midwife?*, *About yourself* can be very effective in making the questionnaire user-friendly. They explain and set up explanations, helping to take the participant from thinking about one type of information to the next.
- Put the questions in an order which is logical and meaningful to the participant. You can analyse and present the results in any order relevant to your research objectives.
- Be clear about the instructions for answering each question, such as *circle the response which most closely resembles your own* or *tick ONE box only*.
- Give a clear explanation of what the questionnaire is about, what it will be used for and a reason, meaningful to the respondent, about why they should complete the form. The title does not have to be that of your research project: use the title as a hook to get attention and gain the interest of the participant.
- Make use of a range of font styles, type sizes, bold, italic and underlining to help the participant through the form.
- Start with an easy response to gain interest and compliance.
- Move from the general to the specific.
- Place critical questions about a third of the way through; participants have warmed to the subject but have not yet become bored or impatient with it.
- Say thank you at the end.
- Be explicit about what to do with the completed form, even if you include a return envelope; this could be mislaid, so you should repeat the return instructions, including the address at the end of the form (see Box 15.5).

Box 15.5 Example of instructions for completed questionnaire

Thank you for giving us your views. Your time and effort is very much appreciated.

Please return this form to: *Gillian Wright, Health Care Research Unit, Freepost, University of Bradford.*
You do not need to use a stamp.

Piloting the questionnaire

How do you know if the questionnaire will work? The pilot is simply a trial of the questionnaire to see how the questions work in practice. It is best to start this process by asking colleagues to complete the form and then perhaps non-colleagues. This will highlight any obvious problems. You would then move on to asking a small number of people who will be typical of your sample to consider the questionnaire.

The most effective way to pilot is, not simply to ask people to read through the form, but to ask them to complete it as if they were a respondent. Then ask them what worked well and what did not work for them. Even with a small number of pilot returns, you can begin to enter the responses into a data file. This is an important element of this process. It will highlight any question structures which are difficult to enter, analyse and interpret. It may also show any layout issues which will help with data input; for example, numbering responses (scales are an obvious example) helps you to translate the answers into data.

A REALISTIC APPROACH

Questionnaires can never be perfect for everyone. The aim is to facilitate generalization about the behaviour and attitudes of different groups of people and, to this end, a questionnaire enables you to ask a large number of people the questions in exactly the same way. Some questions will work better than others. Some people will be able to answer more easily than others. You may have to ask a number of related questions to address complex or emotive issues. A questionnaire will give you a snapshot. Remember that the environment changes, services change, people change. The information from a questionnaire will not last forever. It will give you insight into your sample to facilitate communication and service provision that has a relevance to the identified needs and wants of your community.

FURTHER READING

Bell J 'Designing and Administering Questionnaires' in Bell J *Doing your research project* Milton Keynes: Open University; 1996

Oakley A *Doing Feminist Research* London: Routledge; 1981

Schuman H, Presser S *Questions and Answers in Attitude Surveys* London: Sage; 1998

de Vaus AD 'Constructing Questionnaires' in Bell J *Administering Questionnaires* Milton Keynes: Open University; 1996

16

Conducting interviews with individuals and groups

Sally Marchant and Natalie Kenney

KEY ISSUES

- Why conduct an interview study?
- Different types of interview
- Advantages and disadvantages of using interviews
- A guide to conducting an interview
- The role of the midwife

INTRODUCTION

Interview studies are undertaken when the researcher wants to understand how people view their world and their life, what their opinions and thoughts are about certain issues, topics, attitudes or behaviours. The researcher aims to understand the world from the participant's point of view. Interviews are widely used in research in midwifery and have helped to answer many important questions about midwifery and the delivery of maternity care, for example, exploring midwives' attitudes and perceptions, obtaining the views of women using the maternity services or evaluating the maternity services.

WHY CONDUCT AN INTERVIEW STUDY?

- Interviews are useful in *forming* or *generating a hypothesis*, particularly when little is known of the area being researched.
- Interviews can be used to *test existing hypotheses*.
- Interviews are a beneficial precursor to questionnaire studies as they can help to establish the *terminology* and *definitions* commonly used by the target population, as well as identifying the *variety of views* and *opinions* about certain topics.
- Interviews are a valuable method to use when researching *sensitive topics* as participants may be reluctant to record sensitive information on a questionnaire. An interview may elicit more information as the participant may feel more comfortable once a friendly rapport has been established.

- Interviews are useful when researching *complicated topics* as they allow for the extent of the complexity to emerge.

Types of interview

There are a variety of ways in which interview methods can be used. Each method is capable of providing the researcher with different levels of information, but the type of interview used will depend on the research question being asked.

The *structured interview* requires some knowledge of the subject matter being studied as predetermined questions are usually asked in the same order to all participants. This allows for statistical comparisons to be made between those taking part. The data obtained may lack depth as a limited number of responses are usually provided to the often *closed questions*, but this can make it easier to code the responses and analyse the data. There is not much scope for the participant to discuss or for researchers to record issues not contained within the interview schedule and valuable information about the subject may not be obtained. Structured interviews are suited to large sample sizes because answers are standardized and can be easily quantified, which allows for results to be more generalizable to the relevant population.

The structured interview is the best method to use when conducting telephone interviews as the interviews are generally quite short and require a certain amount of structure so that data can be easily recorded. Conducting an interview over the telephone reduces the effect of observable characteristics which may influence the interview process, such as the gender, age, class and ethnicity of the researcher.

Research example

A national survey of maternity units sought information about the numbers of women and the facilities available for women who wanted to labour and/or give birth in water in England and Wales. An initial postal questionnaire to heads of midwifery services was followed up by a structured telephone interview with midwives who had specialist knowledge about local practices and policies to do with labour and/or birth in water (Alderdice et al 1995).

In a *semi-structured interview* the researcher usually asks predefined, often *open-ended questions* about certain themes, but not necessarily in the same order. Prompt questions may be asked to explore a certain area in more detail based upon the answers provided by the respondent. This type of questioning allows the respondents to discuss issues or topics which they feel are relevant to the subject but which may not be contained in the interview schedule, allowing for a greater exploration of the topic under study. This method of interviewing also allows the researcher to adapt the interview to the participant's level of understanding about the research topic.

Research example

A descriptive survey of the expectations and experiences of postnatal women over the first 12 weeks following the birth was undertaken using semi-structured interviews to explore these issues with women. Where sensitive questions were being asked the use of 'prompt cards' with coded responses were used. Subsequent semi-structured questionnaires were used to complete the survey (Marchant & Garcia 1993, Marchant 1995).

The *in-depth interview* is effective if researchers have very limited knowledge of the area being studied. They are useful to develop ideas or research the initial hypothesis. The in-depth interview usually begins with the researcher asking an open-ended question about the topic of study with the intention that the participant will then give an account of their own viewpoint. The researcher may pose further questions to the participant to explore a certain area in more detail or to clarify a particular response. Owing to the large amount of data generated and the time spent analysing data, in-depth interviews usually have small sample sizes. This can make it difficult to generalize the findings, but the researcher will gain a more in-depth understanding of the topic.

Research example

In-depth interviews were conducted with 11 women which aimed to examine their experiences of labour and the birth of their baby. The interviews revealed that these women placed great trust in their midwives' expertise and knowledge, which may have an effect on the relationship between a woman and her midwife; also that the women wanted an active part in the control of their labour but were not always sure about how to communicate their needs to the midwife (Bluff & Holloway 1994).

Focus groups generate data through the interactions of a particular group which has been brought together by the researcher to discuss a particular subject or theme. They are used as a research method to enhance the development, testing and application of research theories. They are particularly relevant where the topic is of a very specific nature, or involves only part of a population. A structured or pre-determined framework may be used by the facilitator of the group, or the discussion may be completely without structure. The use of a pre-determined framework is debatable in its effect on enhancement or inhibition of the ideas, opinions and experiences of the group members to be shared and explored. Focus groups can also offer the researcher an insight into the formation of social opinions.

Research example

A survey identified the range for normal duration, colour and amount of vaginal loss after childbirth, and a case control study identified a number of factors associated with postnatal problems of excessive or prolonged vaginal bleeding or uterine infection. Postnatal women were then invited to attend focus groups to discuss the use of this information in the development of information leaflets for use by postnatal women following delivery. The focus groups followed a predetermined framework based on the findings of the survey and case control study, and the discussion from the group brought out the views of the women in relation to the use of this information in practice (Marchant et al in press, Marchant et al unpublished).

Advantages and disadvantages of conducting interviews

Advantages

- Interviews generally produce a high response rate.
- Both researcher and participant can clarify any misunderstood questions or responses.
- Questions are less likely to be left unanswered.
- With semi-structured and in-depth interviews, the person being interviewed can define their own responses.
- Interviews allow for the complex human experience to emerge such as views, opinions, feelings and experiences.
- Supplementary data may also be obtained, for example, incidents that influenced the interview such as the participant's degree of understanding or their social and behavioural characteristics. This type of information can be useful as non-verbal communication can validate or emphasize certain points that the participant makes in the analysis of the interviews.

Disadvantages

- Interviews tend to be quite expensive to conduct.
- Data collection can be quite time consuming.
- Participants may provide socially acceptable or logical responses, rather than their real emotions or opinions about the topic.
- Data analysis can be time consuming as interviews tend to produce a large amount of data.

- Semi-structured and in-depth interviews generally have a small and selective sample size, due in part to the costs and time associated with them.
- There may be difficulties in replicating the interviews to assess the validity of the results.
- Information obtained from interviews may not always be generalizable.
- The researcher may influence the participant or the direction of the interview in a number of ways which can bias or affect the validity of the data.

A GUIDE TO CONDUCTING A SEMI-STRUCTURED OR AN IN-DEPTH INTERVIEW STUDY

1. Define the research question.
2. Critically *examine the literature* concerning the topic under study:
   - How have similar research topics been conducted?
   - Were the methods chosen in previous studies the best way to conduct those studies?
   - What were the advantages and disadvantages of using these methods in previous studies?
   - What were the findings?
3. Is an interview study the most appropriate way to answer the research question?
   - How much information is already available?
   - Could other research methods answer the question more effectively?
4. Choose the most suitable type of interview to use – structured, semi-structured, in-depth or a focus group.
5. Gain *ethical approval* to conduct study.
6. Determine the *sample size*. Interview studies are usually associated with small sample sizes owing to the time and costs involved. Structured interviews, however, usually require larger sample sizes to increase their generalizability. Interviews tend to produce a vast amount of data which in some cases may make it impractical to conduct a study with a larger sample size. The sample size needed depends entirely on the question being asked. However, it is generally considered that an adequate sample has been obtained if no new themes or ideas appear to be emerging from the data.
7. Formulate the questions to be asked during the interviews. These may be structured or prompt questions. Where possible, use open-ended questions so that the participant can provide spontaneous information. If using a structured questionnaire, questions should be presented in a logical order. Ensure that the terminology used is not ambiguous.
8. Write to the sample population asking them if they would like to

participate in the research study. It is good practice to include the following in the contact letter:

- A clear explanation of the objectives of the research.
- An estimate of how long interviews are expected to last.
- Details of where the interviews are to be conducted.
- Information of any intention to record interviews and in what format, e.g. audio or video.
- A guarantee that responses will be confidential, that respondents will be anonymous in any reports arising from research and that they can withdraw at any time.

9. Conduct a *pilot interview/s* to assess the suitability of the questions being asked.

- Listen to the recordings of the pilot interview/s.
- Are questions being asked in a leading, suggestive or ambiguous manner?
- How can this be minimized in future interviews?
- What effect are you, as a researcher, having on the interview process?
- Transcribe the pilot interview/s and conduct a preliminary analysis of the data – this will enable questions to be further refined for use in future interviews, as well as ensuring that the data emerging will assist in answering the research question.

10. Conduct remaining interviews. Throughout the study, *field notes* should be kept. Field notes can be used to document events which may not be evident from the interview recording and they can be a data source in their own right. They can also be used to document the researcher's own thoughts and feelings about the interviews, as well as documenting any emerging themes which become apparent during the course of the interviews. Interviews should be recorded using either visual or audio aids as this will assist greatly when interpreting and analysing the large amount of data obtained.

11. Transcribe recorded data. It is worthwhile reading over transcribed data whilst listening to the interview recording. Note any errors that may have occurred during transcription. This will ensure that data have been transcribed verbatim and that no valuable data are lost.

12. Analysis of the data. There are a variety of different ways in which interview data can be analysed.

- The development of codes and categories can be applied to narrative data in a quantifying exercise which aids in the management and manipulation of interview data.
- Data can be analysed manually, but this can be a time consuming process.
- There are several different computer software packages available

which can assist with handling and analysing the large amounts of data generated in interviews.

- It is beneficial to have someone to assist with the analysis as this may help to reduce bias.

13. Write up and disseminate interview results.

THE MIDWIFE AS INTERVIEWER

Interview studies are particularly suited to use by midwives who are conducting research. They already have much experience of eliciting information from women throughout the perinatal period. However, there are various issues concerning the clinical midwife who is also assuming a research role which should be addressed before the start of any interview study. In some circumstances, the researcher may experience difficulties in distinguishing between the role of midwife and that of a researcher. As a researcher undertaking an interview study, every effort should be made to avoid influencing the responses of the participant by refraining from offering professional or clinical opinions during the course of the interview (see Chapter 4).

It is helpful at the outset of the study to consider a range of possible situations which may throw up personal or professional dilemmas. For example, think about how to cope with certain attitudes, behaviours or responses or how to resolve conflict without affecting the participant's responses.

Sooi-Ken Too (1996) provides a good example of the problems which she encountered as a midwife doing an interview study with new mothers and midwifery colleagues, and how she dealt with these difficulties. She discusses the dilemmas involved in being supportive and caring to a woman who was distressed about the care she had received, while also trying to avoid influencing the woman or revealing her own feelings and thoughts about the situation. Trying to maintain a non-judgmental and neutral role when interviewing midwifery colleagues was also an issue, particularly when colleagues sought her opinion about whether correct care had been given, or tried to elicit her support for improving the management structure in the maternity unit.

CONCLUSION

Interviews are probably the most familiar and the most commonly used form of research tool. The use of interview methods may appear to be relatively straightforward, but they require attention to detail and rigour to be valid and reliable methods of enquiry. Midwifery practice lends itself well to these methods and the range of topics related to midwifery which could benefit is extensive. We would encourage the appropriate use of these methods in midwifery research, but with an awareness of the time and personal contributions from the participants involved.

FURTHER READING

Basch C 'Focus Group Interviews: an under utilized research technique for improving theory and practice in health education' *Health Education Quarterly* 1987; **14:** 411–8

Kitzinger J 'Focus Groups, method or madness?' in: Boulton M *Challenge and innovation: methodological advances in social research on HIV/AIDS* London: Taylor and Francis; 1994

Kitzinger J 'Introducing focus groups' *British Medical Journal* 1995; **311:** 299–302

Kvale S *Interviews: an introduction to qualitative research interviewing* USA: Sage; 1996

Mathieson A 'Interviewing Techniques' *Nurse Researcher* 1994; **1:** 3

Oakley A 'Interviewing Women: a contradiction in terms' in Roberts H *Doing Feminist Research* London: Routledge and Kegan Paul; 1981

O'Brien K 'Improving Survey Questionnaires Through Focus Groups' in Morgan D *Successful focus groups: advancing the state of the art* London: Sage; 1993

Oppenheim AN *Questionnaire Design, Interviewing and Attitude Measurement* London: Pinter Publishers; 1994

Polit DF, Hungler BP *Nursing Research: Principles and Methods* Fifth edition Philadelphia, USA: JB Lippincott; 1995

Robson C *Real World Research* Part 3 – Tactics – the method of data collection: Interviews and questionnaires Chapter 9. Oxford: Blackwells; 1993

REFERENCES

Alderdice F, Renfrew MJ, Marchant S, Ashurst H, Hughes P, Berridge G, Garcia J 'Labour and Birth in Water in England and Wales: survey report' *British Journal of Midwifery* 1995; **3:** 375–382

Bluff R, Holloway I 'They Know Best: women's perceptions of midwifery care during labour and childbirth' *Midwifery* 1994; **10:** 157–164

Marchant S, Alexander J, Garcia J 'BLIPP2 (Blood Loss in the Postnatal Period) Final Report' Unpublished, NPEU

Marchant S, Garcia J 'The NPEU Postnatal Care Project' in: *Midwives: hear the heartbeat of the future. Proceedings of the International Confederation of Midwives 23rd International Congress Vancouver May 9–14* 1993; **III:** 1171–1180

Marchant S, Alexander J, Garcia J, Ashurst H, Alderdice F, Keene J 'Blood Loss in the Postnatal Period – The BLiPP Study: A survey of women's experiences of vaginal loss from twenty four hours to three months after childbirth' (in press)

Marchant S 'Real Mothers Don't Need to Rest After the Birth of Their Baby' *Maternity Action* 1995; **67:** 8–10

Too SK 'Issues in Qualitative Research: practical experiences in the field' *Nurse Researcher* 1996; **3(3):** 80–91

17

Conducting participant and non-participant observational studies

Natalie Kenney and Sally Marchant

KEY ISSUES

- Using observation in research
- Advantages and disadvantages of using observation
- Sampling and data collection
- The role of the midwife

INTRODUCTION

Observational studies are used to study and record the behaviour, characteristics and interactions of individuals or groups in pre-existing or artificial settings. Observational studies are most commonly used in the generation and development of research theory.

Taken in its broadest form, the work of midwives could be used as an example of observational work, as much of midwifery practice is dependent upon the observation of women and babies. The analysis of such observation is then used to implement or adapt the planned care and the conclusion is an evaluation of the actions taken. Current guidance on reflection in individual and corporate practice builds on this. An example would be the assessment of the condition of the infant at birth and recording the Apgar score. The use of Apgar scores is a well recognized (if debatable) device in research for assessing outcomes.

USING OBSERVATIONAL STUDIES

In the research context, the use of observational studies offers insight into a variety of different aspects of midwifery and maternity care. Observational studies can focus on one particular aspect of behaviour or they may explore a range of behaviours. These might include the following:

- The type and extent of verbal and non-verbal *communications* between those being observed. For example:
  - Observing the interactions which occur between midwives and women during labour (Kirkham 1989, Bergstrom et al 1997).
  - Observing the interactions of midwife childbirth educators and parents taking antenatal classes (Hallgren et al 1994).

- The *characteristics* of those being observed. For example:
  - Observing differences between midwives and new mothers in their perceptions of the needs of new mothers in the first few months following childbirth (Laryea 1989).
- The *clinical conditions* of those being observed. For example:
  - Observing and documenting skin changes and pain in the nipple during the first week of breastfeeding (Ziemer & Pigeon 1993).
  - The measurement of postpartum fundal height by different midwives and the follow-up of women to assess postpartum involution patterns identified differences in practice and in current theory (Cluett 1994, Cluett 1995).
- The *environmental conditions* which may affect the ways people behave. For example:
  - How women used bed curtains in a maternity ward as a way of maintaining privacy, seeking attention or support (Burden 1998).
  - The environment of midwifery care for women of Asian descent (Bowler 1993).
- The *activities* of those being observed. For example:
  - Observing how midwives provide routine care for women experiencing normal deliveries in a particular area (Maimbolwa et al 1997).
  - How midwives perform sterile vaginal examinations (Bergstrom et al 1992).
- The *skills* of those being observed. For example:
  - Determining the extent to which midwives take the initiative to establish early breastfeeding (Garforth & Garcia 1989).
- *changes in behaviour* during a certain time period.
  - Observing changes in the teaching skills of antenatal teachers, midwives and health visitors before and after attendance on a teaching course (Murphy-Black 1991).

Participant observation

In participant observational studies the researcher takes on a functional and participatory role in the setting being observed, being at once both researcher and midwife. There are two types of participatory role which the researcher can undertake:

1. Those being observed are aware that research is being undertaken and of the role which the researcher is playing. It has been suggested that the researcher who undertakes a participant observer role minimizes the effect they have upon those being observed. The researcher is seen to be involved in what he or she is also observing (Polit & Hungler 1995).

2. In some studies knowledge of the role of the researcher, or knowledge

of the research agenda, would substantially alter the behaviour of those being observed. In such cases participants might not be informed about the role of the researcher, or even about what is being observed. There are ethical and methodological issues which arise from this approach. Where the researcher takes a completely participant role, regardless of whether the research focus is known to the group, they may become so involved in that role that it becomes difficult to adhere to the research agenda or to extract themselves and their findings from the group. Where neither the researcher or the research focus is revealed to the participants, situations may arise where the researcher is required to abandon the research in response to clinical need.

Non-participant observation

In non-participant observational studies the researcher does not take an active part in the setting being observed. There are two types of non-participant observation:

1. The researcher remains visible to those being observed but maintains a distance from the events going on and does not interact with those being observed. This type of study could pose both moral and ethical problems if the researcher is approached by those being observed and encouraged to take an active role, or if it appears to the researcher that her knowledge and expertise are required. This type of study might influence the way in which people behave if they are aware that they are being observed, known as the *Hawthorne effect*. However, it has been suggested that once participants become used to the researcher's presence they begin to display more normal behaviour.

2. The researcher is not known or visible to those being observed. The participants may or may not be aware that they are participating in a research project. For instance, the researcher observes events through a two-way mirror. The findings obtained from this type of observational study are limited as the researcher does not engage in events or interact with informants, so the situation being observed may be misinterpreted.

When undertaking non-participant observation with mothers and babies, in line with professional accountability the researcher would intervene if there is a risk to either mother or baby.

ADVANTAGES AND DISADVANTAGES OF OBSERVATIONAL STUDIES

Advantages

- Observational studies can help to overcome the differences between what people *say* they might do in a particular situation, and what they *actually* do when in that situation.

- A researcher undertaking an observational study may notice behaviours which the participants had, themselves, been unaware of.
- Observational studies can be enhanced by utilizing a number of different types of information gathering processes, for instance interviews, informal discussions, case notes, medical records, letters, pictures and other images.
- They are also a useful method to use with other research methods such as interviews and questionnaires to gain a complete picture of the phenomena being studied.

Disadvantages

- There is usually a high rate of refusal to participate in an observational study.
- Initially, it may be difficult to gain access to and establish a rapport with those being observed.
- There is a risk that those being observed will exhibit distorted behaviour if they are aware that they are being observed.
- Ethical difficulties may be encountered, for instance, deciding whether to inform those to be observed that you are conducting the study.
- It may be difficult for the researcher to separate professional and research roles.
- Observational studies can be mentally, emotionally and physically exhausting for the researcher.
- Observational studies may be susceptible to observer bias.

SAMPLING

The sample population in observational studies is usually selected to represent a particular group which the researcher is aiming to study. There are two sampling methods commonly used to obtain representative data and these can often be combined:

1. *Time sampling* identifies periods of time during which the events being observed take place. A hypothetical situation might be to observe the time spent by midwives on non-clinical tasks. By using time periods of eight 5 minute intervals over 1 hour, it would be possible to note the activities of the midwives in either a structured or unstructured format.

2. *Event sampling* selects pre-specified events which might be overlooked or missed if a time-sampling framework was used. An example of this might be observing the interaction between a midwife and the breastfeeding mother. The event would be the time during which the baby

was breast fed. When using event sampling it may be preferable to use a structured format as there may be too much detail to record everything that occurs. As an example, the following might be recorded: the proximity of the midwife to the mother, eye contact between midwife and mother, how often or whether the midwife touches the mother or the baby, or how often the midwife speaks to the mother.

DATA COLLECTION

Observational data can be collected in either an unstructured or structured format. *Unstructured observations* are useful if a complete understanding of the complexities of a setting are needed and they are more suited to studies where little is known of the area being observed. They are, therefore, useful in developing hypotheses. Unstructured observational studies are, however, more susceptible to observer bias.

Structured observations have a pre-prepared form on which the researcher is able to record the occurrence of specific events or behaviours. The structured format usually contains certain categories or themes that are known to occur in that setting and which lends this type of observational study to more quantitative analysis. It is good practice to provide space for the documentation of other events or behaviours which may not have been evident at the time of designing the form. Before beginning a structured observational study it is important that explicit definitions of each category are formulated and that these are made known to all of the observers taking part. Structured observational studies are suited to testing existing hypotheses.

Data collection is not limited to the interactions or behaviours of those being observed. Other information which is useful to collect includes:

- Details about the physical setting or environment, for instance a descriptive account or map of the labour ward in which interactions between midwives and women are observed (a prestructured time series is often used).
- Details about the people being observed, for instance, the age, ethnicity or mannerisms of those being observed.
- The amount of observations made and the duration of the observation.
- Other intangible factors related to the setting being observed, including, for example, the effect of visiting hours, meal times or the presence of medical staff upon the setting.

Recording observational data

Data obtained from observational studies are most commonly recorded in field notes. However, they can be recorded with technical assistance such as a video or audio recorder. When using field notes, paper records, or even a hand held dictaphone, it is important that events are recorded as soon as is practically possible, either as the events take place or immediately after the events have occurred, so that valuable information is not lost.

The recording of observational data includes, not only events that actually occur within the setting, but also the researcher's feelings or responses to the event, and perhaps changes in those aspects throughout the duration of the observations.

Data analysis

Analysis of observational data should be done concurrently with the collection of the data. Common to other qualitative data analysis, observational data analysis usually involves the development of codes and categories. Structured observational studies may be analysed quantitatively.

Observer bias

Observer bias can be introduced into the observational study in a number of ways, particularly if the researcher becomes over-familiar with the setting being observed. For example, the knowledge, experience, preconceptions, interest or emotional involvement of the researcher may obscure or distort what is really happening within the setting being observed, leading to incorrect assumptions being made. The researcher may also lose her objectivity in recording certain observations.

To reduce the effect that the researcher may have upon the setting being observed, it is helpful to look for changes in people's behaviour and listen to comments that are relayed back during the course of the study. If, as a result of the observations, there appear to be changes in the way people behave, then the observer may be having an effect on the setting. Using actions and comments such as these to identify the impact of the researcher upon the research setting will help to identify the effect of these upon the research.

MIDWIFE AS OBSERVER

Discussion surrounding the issues of the role of midwife as researcher have been touched upon throughout this chapter; however, the topic warrants further coverage.

It is useful, before beginning any observational study, particularly if colleagues are being observed in practice, to be clear about the extent to which the researcher will participate. For example, if observing the interaction of midwives and women in labour, the extent to which the researcher will support the woman or assist the midwife should be clarified.

Once a decision has been made as to how far the researcher will be involved, every effort should be made to adhere to this, so that the research is not compromised.

The clothes that the researcher wears can influence the interactions between the researcher and the setting being observed. For example, wearing a uniform may help the researcher to blend into the group being observed and may make them appear less of an outsider. On the other hand, however, wearing a uniform in the delivery suite may pose problems by drawing the researcher into assisting in areas which were to be observed.

CONCLUSION

Within midwifery, observational studies can provide a rich source of knowledge about aspects of maternity care from the perspective of both care-givers and women. The in-depth approach of this research method, particularly for areas concerning emotional, psychological and sensitive issues, will enhance midwifery practice by informing midwives of the range of possible responses in various settings. With this in mind, research using this method may pose ethical dilemmas and there is a need for awareness of the possible effect upon those being observed. In an attempt to counteract preconceived notions of 'what women want' or 'what midwives should do', observational research is of enormous value. By observing the sense made by women and midwives in their various settings and making this knowledge available, the provision of midwifery care should become more sensitive to the needs of women using the maternity services and those providing care.

FURTHER READING

Gerrish K 'Being a "Marginal Native": dilemmas of the participant observer' *Nurse Researcher* 1997; **5(1)**: 25–34
A personal account of a researcher's experiences of conducting a participant observational study. It describes the benefits, problems and challenges encountered by the researcher when observing nursing colleagues.
Hunt S, Symonds A *The Social Meaning of Midwifery* London: Macmillan; 1995
This is an excellent account of a non-participant observational study conducted on the labour ward, which describes in detail the benefits and problems of doing this type of research study.
Kirkham M 'Midwives and Information Giving in Labour' in Robinson S, Thomson A M *Midwives, Research and Childbirth* 1989; Vol 1. Chapter 6. 117–138
This chapter comprehensively describes the conduct of a research project using observation as the main method in a clinical setting. The collection of data using written record sheets is described and the problems of undertaking research in a clinical area is documented.
Mathieson A 'Observation' *Nurse Researcher* 1994; **2(2)**
This edition of the journal contains a number of articles about the practicalities of conducting observational studies.
Mays N, Pope C 'Observational Research Methods in Health Care Settings' *British Medical Journal* 1995; **311**: 182–184

The third in a series of articles on qualitative research within the health care setting, this article provides a good introduction to conducting observational research.
Methven R 'Recording an Obstetric History or Relating to a Pregnant Woman? A study of the antenatal booking interview' in Robinson S, Thomson AM *Midwives, Research and Childbirth* vol 1; 1989
This research combines an observational study of booking interviews and use of semi-structured interviews and questionnaires.

REFERENCES

Bergstrom L, Roberts J, Skillman L, Seidel J '"You'll feel me touching you, Sweetie": Vaginal Examinations during the second stage of labour' *Birth* 1992; **19(1):** 10–18
Bergstrom L, Seidel J, Skillman-Hull L, Roberts J '"I gotta push. Please let me push!" Social interactions during the change from first to second stage labor' *Birth* 1997; **24(3):** 173–180
Bowler IMW 'Stereotypes of Women of Asian Descent in Midwifery: some evidence' *Midwifery* 1993; **9:** 7–16
Burden B 'Privacy or Help? The use of curtain positioning strategies within the maternity ward environment as a means of achieving and maintaining privacy, or as a form of signalling to peers and professionals in an attempt to seek information or support' *J Advanced Nursing* 1998; **27:** 15–23
Cluett ER 'An investigation into the intra rater and inter rater variability of the postpartum abdominal measuring of the distance between the symphisis pubis and the uterine fundus using a paper tape measure: and a longitudinal study of the natural history of uterine involution as described by this measurement' *Unpublished MSc thesis* Guildford: University of Surrey; 1994
Cluett ER, Alexander J, Pickering RM 'Is Measuring Postnatal Symphysis-fundal Distance Worthwhile?' *Midwifery* 1995; **11:** 174–83
Garforth S, Garcia J 'breastfeeding Policies in Practice – "No wonder they get confused"' *Midwifery* 1989; **5:** 75–83
Hallgren A, Kihlgren M, Norberg A 'A Descriptive Study of Childbirth Education Provided by Midwives in Sweden' *Midwifery* 1994; **10:** 215–224
Kirkham M 'Midwives and Information-giving During Labour' in Robinson S, Thomson AM *Midwives, Research and Childbirth* Vol 1; 1989
Laryea M, 'Midwives' and Mothers' Perceptions of Motherhood' in Robinson S, Thomson AM *Midwives, Research and Childbirth* Vol 1; 1989
Maimbolwa MC, Ransjö-Arvidson AB, Ng'andu N, Sikazwe N, Diwan VK 'Routine Care of Women Experiencing Normal Deliveries in Zambian Maternity Wards: a pilot study' *Midwifery* 1997; **13:** 125–131
Murphy-Black T 'Antenatal Education: evaluation of a post-basic training course' in Robinson S, Thomson AM *Midwives, Research and Childbirth* Vol 2; 1991
Polit DF, Hungler BP *Nursing Research: Principles and Methods* Fifth edition, Philadelphia: JB Lippincott Company; 1995
Ziemer MM, Pigeon JG 'Skin Changes and Pain in the Nipple During the 1st Week of Lactation' *JOGGN* 1993; **22(3):** 247–256

Index